WHY DIDN'T

Why Didn't They Listen?

Renata Payne

SilverWood

Published in 2015 by the author
using SilverWood Books Empowered Publishing®

SilverWood Books Ltd
30 Queen Charlotte Street, Bristol, BS1 4HJ
www.silverwoodbooks.co.uk

ISBN 978-1-78132-328-1 (paperback)
ISBN 978-1-78132-329-8 (ebook)

British Library Cataloguing in Publication Data
A CIP catalogue record for this book is available from
the British Library

Set in Adobe Garamond Pro by SilverWood Books
Printed on responsibly sourced paper

For Ellie and Carl

I am profoundly grateful for the steadfast support I have received
from the many family members, friends and colleagues, past and
present, who truly believe in my professional competence
and integrity.

From the cowardice that shrinks from new truth
From the laziness that is content with half-truth
From the arrogance that thinks it knows all truth
O God of Truth, deliver us.

Ancient Prayer

Contents

Introduction

Imagine that a fifty-three-year-old businessman goes to his GP complaining that recently his memory has become worse, he can't concentrate, he's made a mess of his tax returns for the first time ever, and his wife is losing patience because he can't manage the DIY that he's been doing for years. He would expect the doctor to find out what was wrong.

The main things the doctor would have in mind are dementia, depression and drinking too much alcohol. Any of them could be the cause or an effect. The doctor would address the problem by asking about his drinking, checking for life events that might be making him depressed, for symptoms specific to depression, and make an initial assessment of his intellectual (known as cognitive) difficulties.

The reason for the assessment isn't to make an on-the-spot diagnosis: it is to provide a baseline. The next step would be to check the effect of an anti-depressant on the symptoms, especially the presenting complaints, and deal with the role of alcohol, if any. The doctor might organise liver function and other blood tests. The input of a close associate of the patient, if available, is important because, in neurological and psychological illnesses especially, it can differ significantly from that of the patient.

After six months to a year, if the position is still unclear or there has been no improvement in the symptoms, he should be referred to the local specialist. Both mild cognitive impairment and dementia in a fifty-three-year-old man need full investigation to exclude fully treatable causes (e.g. thyroid disorders and some vitamin deficiencies), conditions needing aggressive treatment (e.g. brain tumours) and deal with remediable vascular (blood supply) risk factors like high blood pressure, dyslipidaemias (e.g. raised cholesterol) and diabetes. This may slow the progress of the condition and prevent further dementia due to strokes.

This is what should have happened. In Carl Valente's case it did not. He was taken on his first visit to his GP down the wrong diagnostic road – depression. The GP continued on it despite warning signs from the patient, his wife, and other close associates that he needed to turn back. And the repeated warnings of his inner satnav, his medical training, to turn around when possible i.e. refer the patient to a specialist. If only he'd had it switched on.

That was how the tragedy became a nightmare.

PART 1

On Carl

Why didn't they listen?

1

When bad things happen

Bad things happened to Carl and Ellie. If, as they say, humour is based on reversal of expectations we ought still to be laughing now, a decade after the end of their story.

Except we're not laughing. The dementia that would slowly kill Carl was always going to be a tragedy. And the tragedy became a nightmare when, for three years, they were given no explanation. Even left feeling they themselves were to blame.

Their right to plan their own lives before dementia took hold had been denied. Their best opportunities for enjoying whatever moments of happiness remained for them had been lost. They were replaced by marital friction as his behaviour grew ever crazier without his wife knowing why, despite repeated attempts to get their doctor to respond to her entreaties and her husband's complaints. They were replaced for her by frantic overwork settling his massive business debts, keeping her business, their home and livelihood going, and caring for him as he regressed into toddlerhood.

Things like this – and worse – are still happening. To little people like this couple who don't count in a big society although they are what makes a big society.

They are from poor backgrounds where you had to struggle to make ends meet, sometimes even to stay alive. Education was for those who lived in a different world and whom you wouldn't meet. Apart from your doctor.

But they had these priceless assets: raw talent, energy,

dependability and humanity. You could trust them with your life.

Together they'd built their own home surrounded by an acre of beautiful garden from which she ran an upmarket B&B while he'd established a wholesale butchery some years previously. They'd seen their two sons come out of university with good degrees, marry and present them with grandchildren. Life had been good.

Until that phone call.

2

'What's happening, Ellie?'

The phone call that will change Ellie's life forever comes on a hot August afternoon in 1990.

'It's Arthur here. Can you come over? It's about Carl's tax figures.'

'I'm very busy, Arthur. You know what the B&B's like in the summer. Shall I get Carl to ring you?'

'I need to see *you*. I don't understand it,' he says.

She drives the five miles to his office. Has Carl been cooking the books, she wonders. Surely not. Okay, things have been hard in butchery in recent years with the red meat and cholesterol problem, mad cow disease, and supermarkets undercutting local wholesale butchers by using foreign suppliers.

And next year's health and safety legislation[1] on abattoirs means that Carl will be faced with either an expensive upgrade of his wholesale butchery premises or downsize to retailing of locally sourced quality produce. But he's always been adaptable, and never sought huge profits so the idea of him cooking the books is unthinkable.

Arthur is seated at his desk when she arrives.

'Look at this!' he says, pointing to a figure circled in red, 'He's put down £2,000,000 profit. That's so ridiculous it beggars belief.'

So Carl can't be cooking the books, Ellie thinks. The page of figures Arthur shows her has nearly as much accountant's red ink on as Carl's blue. It looks like one of those pages of homework that got you one out of ten and a 'See me!' note off the teacher.

Arthur didn't know, although Ellie will always wonder if he'd had his suspicions, that, at the age of fifty-three, dementia was killing the thinking part of Carl's brain, a few cells at a time. That's why he was incapable of providing the figures needed for his tax returns.

Over the next thirteen years dementia would kill, piecemeal, the entire mind and spirit of the man who was Carl, taking him back through the stages of childhood until only the primitive parts of the brain controlling bodily functions remained. At the age of sixty-six, even these remnants of him would be dead.

'What's happening, Ellie?' Arthur asks.

She shakes her head. I can't understand it, she thinks. There haven't been any problems with Carl's accounts before. He'd always had a good head for figures. He'd even begun an accountancy course himself after he left school.

He'd given it up because he couldn't bear the thought of sitting at a desk all day for the rest of his working life. He'd become a manager for a large wholesale butcher with twenty men under him before setting up his own wholesale butchery supplying meat to one of the large supermarkets and employing six people.

Images of a changed Carl are crowding her mind. They've got problems with his mother who'd had another stroke, tenants from Hell in the flats, and they've recently had to put Judy, his favourite dog, down. He'd always been a workaholic, taking these things in his stride, but he'd started coming home earlier in the evenings. He'd get a beer from the fridge, sit down in the armchair and continue drinking.

Okay, she thinks, Carl's always been good company, enjoyed a drink or several with friends or family. That was all, though. She'd never known him drink on his own like this. And sometimes in the evenings when he was sitting quietly watching TV, she'd see tears running down his cheeks. But he'd clam up if she tried to probe.

She glances at Arthur. He's looking puzzled and sad. They'd first met during Carl's teenage years when Arthur, a trainee accountant in his twenties, was his parents' lodger. After Carl's father died of a heart attack when Carl was only twenty-one, Arthur had become something of a father figure.

Admit it, she tells herself, there's something wrong with Carl.

'I'll see he goes to the doctor,' she tells Arthur.

Carl sees the doctor in August 1990, a date she will never forget.

He comes home afterwards saying he's been told overwork and their other problems are making him anxious and depressed, and he should cut down on his drinking. He's been given some tablets and a relaxation tape to help him cope.

Good job I made him see the doctor, Ellie thinks, he'll soon be all right.

Carl stops drinking, she's sure of that, and he doesn't seem sad any more. He goes back a couple of times for check-ups.

But he still isn't right.

He'd always enjoyed helping with the B&B. Anything from DIY to looking after the guests and often helping with the breakfasts before going to work. She can depend on him. They're a good team. Guests come back again and again and give excellent feedback for the tourist guides. During university graduation week they're always fully booked and run off their feet, afterwards sitting back and enjoying the satisfaction of a job well done.

Over the next six months Carl keeps making mistakes that you can only get away with once in a while. Word soon gets round, and if it does then the B&B will be deleted from the guides and she'll eventually be out of business.

One morning she asks him to take a kipper up to the guest in Room One. Room One, Carl. Don't forget. She always has to remind him these days. He gets as far as the kitchen door and asks her which room.

'Room One, Carl, Room One! Why don't you listen?'

He goes upstairs and returns without the kipper.

Phew! she thinks.

Until the guest who'd ordered it rings down to ask where his kipper is. Oh, no! Carl must have taken it to Room Five. She rushes in to be greeted by a plate bearing a few clean fish bones, and a happy guest who tells her not to worry about it. He hasn't had a kipper for ages and he really enjoyed it, thank you. No problem.

But there is a problem. It's her last kipper, she's sure. She's expecting a delivery from the smokehouse later. She'll have to find an alternative for the guest who'd ordered it.

She decides to check in the freezer just in case there's one left. Carl is hovering behind her. She can't get past.

'Carl! Get out of my way!' she shouts. He looks at her with a beaten-dog expression just like Judy's if they'd shouted at her. Then without saying anything he goes into the sitting room. She wants to put her arms round him, say it doesn't matter.

But it does matter. She's landed with placating the guest in Room One. Or he might not come again. He's a regular. She can't afford to lose him.

The kipper isn't an isolated incident.

Carl keeps directing guests to the wrong rooms. Anything from showing them into already occupied rooms to getting double and twin-room guests mixed up. They might accept the mistake for the first night but they'll expect a change-over the next day. That means explanations, apologies, beds to change, rooms to clean, extra sheets to launder to keep guests happy and the business afloat.

Carl's salesman, who often drops in, tells Ellie they're concerned about him at work, saying he's lost his grip on things.

His mistakes are driving her frantic with worry and exhaustion; he says the trouble is her nagging and perfectionism. She wonders what he's telling the doctor. Thanks, Doc, I'm miles better on those tablets you gave me – words she can imagine rolling off his tongue.

And the new regulations requiring major alterations to the workplace come into force soon: it's either that at a cost of thousands or switch to retail.

He's always adapted to change before, Ellie thinks. But is he up to it now, she wonders. Maybe he'd be better off just selling his business and running the B&B with me. That would take all the stress off him. But we've never interfered before in each other's business. And how do I know he isn't going to get better once the doctor's found out what's wrong. How would I feel then, she wonders.

I'd better see the doctor myself, she thinks. Let him know what's really happening. She's in a long time explaining how it's affecting their marriage and both businesses at a critical time. How at fifty-three he's begun acting like he was three or eighty-three and getting worse not better. The doctor seems to listen.

She comes away believing that he will see Carl and get him back to his old self.

3

'I was looking at a mountain'

– Ellie Valente

By autumn 1991 Ellie begins to wonder if the change to retail butchery hasn't progressed beyond what seemed like a good idea. Although Carl saw the doctor not long after she did, he hasn't shown any signs of improvement.

He comes home from work at lunchtimes and doesn't go back. Previously excellent DIY skills like putting up curtain rails defeat him. He gets lost on local roads, saying there must have been a diversion or they'd changed the junction or made a new one-way system.

After Christmas when she has to see the GP about a minor problem herself, she uses the opportunity to tell him again that she is still worried about Carl. She's given a two week course of a tranquilliser.

In March 1992, worry over what might be happening to Carl's business overcomes her loyalty to him. She asks their son, a finance analyst who lives two hundred miles away, to come home and look at Carl's business accounts. With wages and overheads to pay, the business is losing money at the rate of £700 per week, and Ellie is looking at a debt mountain fifty thousand pounds high.

So, about a year-and-a-half after giving Arthur, the accountant, the figure of £2,000,000 for his profits, there is no hope for the business. They are now dependent on the B&B not only to provide them with a living but also to repay the debts.

*

Carl sees the GP soon afterwards. Over the next year he sees the doctor regularly to get sick notes for anxiety-depression while his behaviour gets worse. Ellie's life consists of drudgery as she pays off the debts, and damage limitation in the B&B caused by Carl's help that's a hindrance. She complains to the GP again about Carl's stupid behaviour. He puts her on Prozac, gives her a relaxation tape and refers her for counselling. Now they both have a relaxation tape and are on and off medication for Carl's undiagnosed dementia.

One day in the summer of 1993, three years after their accountant asked Ellie what was happening, Carl comes home after picking up his sick note.

Ellie reads it.

'He's got to be kidding,' she says.

It's a Return to Work note.

4

'I've had it up to here'

'Carl, do you think you're fit to work?' Ellie asks.

'No!' says Carl, the workaholic.

It's only three weeks, Ellie thinks, since he messed up wiring a plug. He could have killed somebody. It was child's play to him once.

She wonders what that psychologist he saw once or twice in the past three months had been playing at. Carl says she didn't want to see him again because he's managing with reminder lists. I'd have told her a different story, thinks Ellie. Anyway, it's only when people get older they have to write things down that they mustn't forget. Carl's only fifty-six. He's always had a brilliant memory.

What are these professionals doing, she wonders. She phones Dr Bromwich. He says he's been giving Carl sick notes for a long time and can't continue to do so.

This doesn't make sense to Ellie. Whatever was wrong with Carl when Arthur phoned her is still wrong with him now, only more so. She says she doesn't know what they'd make of him at the Job Centre because he isn't fit to work. He'd be a dangerous liability in any job.

Dr Bromwich says she'll have to explain that to a DSS doctor. Ellie phones the DSS. They say that they can't send one of their doctors out at the request of a claimant. It's the GP's job to issue sick notes. If she isn't satisfied, she should complain to the health authority.

I can't do that, she thinks, when I've been with this practice since I was born. But I've had it up to here with all these professionals. After some thought, she demands a visit from the Head of Practice, Dr Stratford.

He listens to both of them then turns to her: 'Your husband needs a brain scan. I'll get him an early appointment with the specialist, Dr White.'

And only six days after Carl's regular GP issued the Return to Work note, he writes out a sick note for eight weeks and hands it to her.

She stands up.

'It's okay. I'll see myself out,' he says.

She's hardly had time to draw breath before she hears the scrunch of his car tyres on the gravel drive.

Thank you, God, Ellie thinks, for this doctor who's done in ten minutes what three years of combined effort didn't. Neither she nor Carl has seen Dr White, the specialist, before but she's heard nothing but good about her from anyone who has – no matter who they are.

Every night until the appointment Ellie prays that Dr White will be able to sort Carl out.

His appointment comes two months later. Although there's a long queue of patients waiting, Dr White listens to both of them, just as if she has all the time in the world. She examines Carl thoroughly, and orders a brain scan plus some other tests.

When they see her again, she says the scan shows Carl hasn't got a brain tumour, but she'll need to keep a close eye on him to be certain of what's going on. Meanwhile she'd like to try him on a drug that often helps with memory problems. It shouldn't be long before they notice an improvement.

That night, reminding herself that it's wrong to expect miracles, Ellie thanks God for this specialist who listens and cares.

5

Freda

One night, about a month after Carl started the tablets, Ellie's phone rings.

Newsnight is almost finished and she's thinking about going to bed.

She wonders who on earth it can be. She doubts if it's anyone wanting to book in at this time of night. I must have forgotten to switch the phone to Sorry, No Vacancies, she thinks. Better answer it, I suppose.

'Hello,' she says after a pause.

'Is that Willowbank House?' asks a man's voice.

'Well, yes, but...'

'It's Tim Jones here from The Red Lion. You know, near the bus station.'

If that's supposed to reassure me, it doesn't, she thinks. She thinks of Saturday night rowdies turning out at closing time, fighting, throwing up all over the pavement and getting themselves into the local paper.

'Have you any vacancies?' he asks.

'Er, well, uh...' she says, giving the game away.

'I'm in a right spot here,' he says, 'I'd better explain.'

He tells her that a distraught, dishevelled woman turned up in the pub about half an hour ago. She'd got off a long distance bus from up north. Said her baby was buried somewhere round here. All she ever wanted to know was where, but nobody would say.

Would've been her twenty-first birthday today, so she said.

And he's stuck here on his own, he says. The wife's had to go over to her mother's or she'd have seen to it.

As wives do, Ellie thinks. She asks him how old the woman is.

'I'd guess in her early fifties,' he says, 'Hard to tell, she's in such a state. I phoned a few people before you and they wouldn't take her. I can't turn her out on a night like this.'

Great! she thinks. Dear God, haven't I got enough problems without you landing me with this? Oh, no! I mustn't think like this when you've sent me Dr White.

I should be grateful, she thinks, that Carl's a lot better now. Only this morning he's managed to lay all the tables properly and take breakfasts into the guests, getting it right with some friendly prompting: 'No, mate, I'm waiting for the full English. The poached egg's for the lady over there.'

She hears a cough on the other end of the line.

'I'm coming for her. Give me about twenty minutes,' she says.

She does a quick room check. Bed made up. Fresh set of fluffy towels and a selection of toiletries in the en-suite. Room cleaned and aired today. TV working. Teabags, coffee and hot chocolate sachets, and biscuit packs on the little table. She fills the small electric kettle with fresh water, turns up the central heating and switches the bedside lamp on. A beam of soft light falls upon the Gideon Bible on the bedside unit.

It'll be warm and cosy by the time we're back, she thinks.

She looks in on Carl. He's fast asleep. It's okay to leave now.

A gust of wind nearly blows the garage door out of her hands. Good job it didn't come off its hinges like that time a few years ago, she thinks to herself. Carl can't mend anything these days.

Inside The Red Lion she finds the publican clearing the tables. They exchange greetings then she goes over to the solitary hunched figure sitting at a table close to the fire, and lays her hand on her arm.

'I'm Ellie,' she tells her. 'I've got a room ready for you.'

The woman gets to her feet. She's about as tall as me, but

29

looks as if she needs feeding up, Ellie thinks.

And she's come with no luggage. Only a big handbag that's seen better days. Never mind that now. Tim's stopped wiping the tables and he's standing looking at them. Waiting for them to leave so he can lock up.

'Let's go, shall we...er...Sorry, I don't know your name,' Ellie says.

'I'm Freda.'

Not much to go on but it could be a local accent.

'Right, Freda. Off we go. It's not far.'

Ellie tells Tim she'll be in touch and they leave The Red Lion. Back home she parks the car and locks it. It can stay outside for one night. It's this poor guest who needs looking after.

'Would you like a drink or a snack before I show you to your room?' Ellie asks once they get inside.

'No, I'll be all right, thanks,' Freda says.

When they go into the room Ellie thinks she sees the tension lines on her guest's face softening. She shows her where everything is.

'Make yourself at home. I'll get you one of my nighties.'

She goes to the linen cupboard in the corridor, returns after a minute and puts a nightdress on the bed.

'I think I'll be able to help you, Freda. We'll get some sleep now and talk about it in the morning. I'll give you a call to see what you'd like for breakfast. Sleep well.'

Ellie goes off to her bed. Carl's fast asleep. Jumbled thoughts chase each other around in her head. Those tablets the specialist gave him seem to be helping a bit – I hope Freda's all right – not knowing where her baby's buried – must have been a stillbirth – it was better than that in Grandma's day – they were poor but they knew how to deal with these things – they helped each other.

Next morning, Ellie's up at six as usual dealing with the guests' breakfasts. She's told Carl about the late arrival last night.

By half past eight she's got everyone fed, cleared the tables and stacked the dishwasher. I'll see to Freda's breakfast now, she thinks.

She phones her room and gets a sleepy 'Hello'. Freda says 'Yes' to a pot of tea brought up to her room, and she couldn't face a mixed grill but a soft boiled egg with a slice of toast would be lovely. Yes, if Ellie's sure it's all right, she'll come down to the kitchen to eat.

Freda appears about half an hour later, stands in the kitchen doorway looking around. Trixie gets up from her basket in the utility room and rushes over wagging her tail.

'Come on in!' Ellie tells her. 'Are you okay with dogs? She'll go back in her basket if I tell her.'

'No, I like dogs.' She bends down to pat Trixie. Carl comes into the kitchen. He smiles and greets Freda.

'Carl,' Ellie says, 'you need to take Trixie for a walk. She hasn't been out yet.'

Carl goes off with Trixie. Ellie turns to Freda.

'I've laid a place for you here,' Ellie says. 'He'll be about three-quarters of an hour. While he's out, I'd better tell you about him.'

She explains that Carl's been getting more forgetful lately. But last month he saw the specialist who is lovely. She's put him on some tablets that seem to be helping but he's still doing silly things at times.

Freda opens her mouth as if to speak but seems to think better of it. Ellie continues: 'Anyway, if he seems to be off-message when you're talking to him, don't worry.'

'It's just that I feel awful,' says Freda, 'landing myself on you when you've got enough problems of your own. And I've got no money left to get back home. I should never have come. But I left in a terrible state.'

She tells Ellie about it between long pauses. Ellie knows how to listen. She was a Samaritans counsellor for years. Freda's keeping the lid on a cauldron of emotions that's threatening to boil over.

Freda had a stillborn baby twenty-one years ago at the local maternity hospital. They wouldn't even let her see the baby, let alone touch her or hold her, before they took her away saying she must forget all about it. She only knew it was a girl because she got an 'Er, yes' to her direct question. Then she was in the post-natal ward for a week, like they were in the sixties and seventies, having to watch all the other mothers feeding their new babies and their visitors coming to admire them.

She saw her doctor and wrote to the hospital a few times, got fobbed off with statements about policy, procedure, confidentiality, and learning to put bad experiences behind her. She and her husband moved up north but they had no children. Every year what would have been her child's birthday to celebrate was a nightmare.

Her first waking thought yesterday was of her child who would have been twenty-one. An independent adult.

She spoke her thoughts. Her husband blew his top. Every year as the day came round it was the same. If she hadn't put it out of her mind by now she was sick. Well, this time he'd had it right up to here.

This time, Freda tells Ellie, she'd had it up to here as well. She had to find her baby. She put on her coat, picked up her handbag, walked out of the house, caught the long distance coach and here she was.

They sit in silence for a few minutes, Freda gazing out of the window at the view of the fields beyond the garden. That's it for now, Ellie thinks. Thank God for the charity that pressured the government to bring in legislation forcing the professionals to do what ordinary people did in her grandma's day.

Ellie looks at the clock. Carl will be back soon.

'Freda,' she says, 'You can stay as long as you need to. The room's free. I've an idea whereabouts in the cemetery they bury the babies from the hospital. They're all together.'

She looks at Freda but her expression doesn't change.

'I'll go and phone the cemetery office,' she says. 'They should be open now.'

She comes back after about fifteen minutes. The babies are buried where she thought – in a peaceful spot under some trees.

She's phoned the vicar on duty: he can fit in a short service there next morning if it would help.

'How do you feel about that, Freda?'

Freda nods, her eyes full of tears. After phoning the vicar back, Ellie comes into the kitchen and puts the kettle on.

'That's done,' Ellie tells her. 'He says to let him know sometime today your feelings about the service, what you'd like, and whether you want him to name her.'

They wake next morning to another crisp, sunny autumn day. After breakfast they go to the cemetery. The vicar is waiting for them in the office. They walk to the babies' burial plot. Ellie and Freda stand side-by-side opposite him.

He conducts the brief service, committing Freda's child to God's safe keeping. A few leaves, red, russet and gold, fall softly through the still air to the ground.

Freda buries her head in Ellie's shoulder and sobs. Ellie and the vicar exchange glances. She mouths to him: 'It's okay.' He comes over to them, places a hand on Freda's arm and says: 'God bless.' Then he goes back to the office.

Ten minutes later, Freda is composed. Ellie picks up the fallen leaves and gives them to her. Freda puts them carefully, gently, into her handbag.

On the way back, Ellie buys Freda's ticket at the bus station, and after lunch sees her off on her journey home.

Two months later, she gets her first Christmas card from Freda.

Fallen Sparrows

Frail humanity prompts grief.
While we mourn
the passing of the old
we can also celebrate a long life.
But a child?
Grief will stifle all other emotions.

In time happy memories
of that brief life
will return,
they will become more precious
but a stillborn child?
Birth and death in one instant
yet that sad single memory
must remain.
No birth should be forgotten
no death should be forgotten.

J.H., 2011

6

'Nail the bastards'

– Carl Valente, 1937–2003

One day next spring Ellie is sitting at the kitchen table with a cup of coffee, feeling completely disconnected.

Two hours ago Carl set off for the clinic alone, saying he could tell them how he was – leaving Ellie behind to nurse her suspicions. If he has turned up, she thinks – not something you can rely on these days – he'll tell whoever he sees how much better he is. They'll say: Keep on taking the tablets. Come back in three months.

She'd wanted to go with Carl and explain that the tablets weren't working as well now. On Bonfire Night, not long after Freda had gone back, he'd let the dog out. Fortunately, they'd managed to coax her back in before she came to any harm. Carl would never have been so careless once. She is worn out with constant worry.

This morning he'd got up early, fumbled about for two hours preparing simple starters for six breakfasts and given them to the wrong people. She could have had the job done herself in a quarter of the time. But he'd have felt useless and unwanted, and blamed her for being a perfectionist and she didn't want that.

If she has to go out, reminding him beforehand to let the answering machine take the phone calls he forgets and tries to do the bookings himself. She returns to a series of muddled and lost messages.

Questions race around her mind. Can I continue living with

this crazy stranger who's taken over Carl's body and is now driving me mad? Can I keep this business, our livelihood, going now that guests are beginning to complain? Can I pay the rest of the debts before they seize the house?

For richer for poorer, for better for worse...marriage vows she'd made thirty-odd years ago but she's too tired to carry on. When she saw the doctor recently wanting a hysterectomy because she was exhausted and severely anaemic he told her they weren't done on the patient's say-so.

In sickness and in health...but will someone ever answer Arthur's question: 'What's happening, Ellie?'

The phone rings.

It's Dr White.

She tells Ellie that, although Carl said he was fine and helping with the B&B, she assessed him as worse. She is phoning, with Carl's permission, to hear Ellie's version.

Someone, Ellie thinks, cares enough about my opinion to go to the trouble of phoning me. She feels like crying but manages to say that she'd wanted to tell Dr White herself that Carl's help was actually a hindrance and driving her mad.

Dr White explains that the brain scan shows cerebral atrophy – his brain has shrunk. That's the cause of his problems. And she should join the Alzheimer's Society because she is going to need a lot of support.

Ellie puts the phone down. The Alzheimer's Society. Bang! So that's it. Dementia. But, she thinks, dementia's something that happens to old people. So it can't be that.

But, really, she knows that it's the truth. Carl's got dementia. Strangely, she feels relieved. They'd both been declared 'Not guilty' after years of worry, and confusion over why, after years of happy marriage, they weren't pulling together any more.

It's all fallen into place, she thinks. The daft things he's been doing. I bet Arthur suspected it with the two million pound profits, and thought I'd be able to enlighten him. All those times I shouted at poor Carl when he couldn't help it. I should have guessed.

But if I should have guessed, the doctor should have known. Known that the problem was inside Carl's head not his business, and not the other way round. It's the doctor's job. You don't expect miracles, but you do expect the truth.

Fat lot of good tablets and relaxation tapes did either of us, she thinks.

We could have gone on the holiday of a lifetime like people do when they're told they've got cancer and I'd have had time to relax for the odd hour in a champagne bubble bath. Instead, every day of the year apart from Christmas, you smile for the guests when your heart is breaking.

Carl comes in.

'How did you get on?' Ellie asks.

'Oh, fine,' he says. He sits down at the table and picks up the paper.

'I'll make us an omelette for lunch,' she says.

After they've eaten, when she asks if he knows what's wrong, he says he doesn't. She says: 'Carl, I'm telling you this for both our sakes. The brain scan shows you've got dementia.'

'Oh!' he gasps.

For the next few minutes he sits gazing out of the window. He seems lost in thought. Then she sees tears coursing down his cheeks.

She makes him a cup of tea, puts it in front of him, and takes him in her arms.

'Carl, what do you want me to do about this?'

He tells her, simply: 'Nail the bastards!'

7

Daffodils

Now they know the diagnosis things are much better between them although Carl is deteriorating in fits and starts. On bad days he can't find fixed objects like the cooker. When Carl undergoes formal psychometric tests, the psychologist is disturbed to find that he is still driving, albeit only on familiar roads. Ellie wonders what the tests would have shown when she first told the doctors her concerns about his driving. She explains that Carl's van is in for its MOT so they'll sell it and she will take sole charge of the keys to their car. Carl never forgives her and grumbles to all his friends about her stopping him driving. Two weeks later Dr Bromwich asks them to come and see him – to explain that Carl probably ought to stop driving.

Fortunately, Ellie manages to finish paying off the debts so she can afford to reduce the number of guests in the B&B and free up more time to devote to Carl's needs. With fewer B&B rooms in use she should qualify for a reduction in her property rating so she asks Dr Bromwich for an open letter on Carl's condition to support her application to the local council's ratings department.

One morning she is reading the paper when a headline catches her eye: DAFFODILS BRING HOPE FOR DEMENTIA SUFFERERS. She reads on:

Trials are beginning in several centres around the country of an extract from wild daffodils and snowdrops called

Galanthamine. These flowers have been used in Eastern European folk remedies for nervous diseases since ancient times but this is the first time a rigorous attempt has been made to test its usefulness in dementia.

Ellie shows Dr Bromwich the cutting. He hasn't heard of the trials or the drug but promises to find out more. I will keep you to that, Ellie thinks.

The doctor is as good as his word. One of the centres is only half-an-hour's drive away. After a series of suitability tests Carl joins the trial the following January. Ellie looks out of the kitchen window at the wild daffodil shoots peeping out of the ground and dares to hope.

Carl's improvement is dramatic. His mood, concentration, memory and practical skills are all better. They both notice it. He gets the breakfast starters right, mows the lawn, digs the garden, and walks the dog every day. Both Dr White and the consultant running the trial find an improvement.

The trial ends after a year and when it does Carl deteriorates. Current UK licencing restrictions make it impossible to obtain more Galanthamine. After having his hopes raised then cruelly dashed, he becomes so depressed that Dr White warns Ellie not to leave him alone. But she must go out sometimes to maintain their home and their livelihood.

It is now spring 1997, four-and-a-half years since Carl first saw the doctor.

Soon afterwards Ellie is again sitting at the kitchen table reading the daily paper when a headline catches her eye: LATEST DRUG HOPE FOR ALZHEIMER'S CASES.

Ellie gives a copy of the article[2] identifying the drug as Aricept to Dr Southam, who replaced Dr Bromwich when he retired recently, and offers to pay for it herself. But, because it is only available on strictly limited licence in the UK, it is the consultant Dr White who, after a struggle, obtains it for Carl on a named patient basis. Luckily, Aricept suits him too and he improves again in both mood and daily activities.

To Daffodils

Fair daffodils, we weep to see
you haste away so soon;
as yet the early-rising sun
has not attained his noon.
Stay, stay
until the hasting day
has run
but to the evensong:
and, having prayed together, we
will go with you along.

We have short time to stay, as you,
we have as short a spring:
as quick a growth to meet decay,
as you, or anything.
We die
as your hours do, and dry
away
like to the summer's rain;
Or, as the pearls of morning's dew,
ne'er to be found again.

Robert Herrick, 1591–1674

8

'I had to do all the chasing'

– A carer

Shortly afterwards, they hear from Dr Southam of a research project looking into the needs of younger people in their area with dementia, including Carl. The survey stemmed from Dr White's wish to do more for local people with early-onset dementia (below the age of sixty-five) who have different needs from the elderly.

They agree to be interviewed by the researcher about their views on the services they received. Through her involvement in the local Alzheimer's Society, Ellie obtains a copy of the report. It is now August 1998.

She is disturbed by what she reads.

The researchers investigated thirty-two local cases, age range twenty-eight to sixty-four at their first visit to their GP. Commenting on the support they received after the formal diagnosis, carers complained that they had to 'do all the chasing to get any help'.

So Ellie wasn't alone. What most disturbed her was that, apart from Carl and two others, the majority had been given a formal diagnosis by around a year after their first visit to the GP. It took three years for Carl – and that was thanks to two other doctors' interventions.

The report noted that the usual reason for late diagnosis was the patient's or the carer's failure to consult their doctor about their difficulties sooner – because they were frightened or in denial. But they also made the point that some clinicians fail to diagnose sooner because nothing can be done until a crisis requires the support services.

Ellie's thoughts are racing.

If Carl had been referred to a specialist after she'd been to see the GP herself about him they'd have closed his business while it was solvent knowing a cure, if there was one, wasn't round the corner. She'd have felt like she was in clover compared with what did happen. She'd sensed at times that the GP saw her as another moaning, menopausal woman, and them both as an uneducated pair who'd swum out of their depth into professional and business circles.

The report stresses the importance of timely diagnosis for, amongst other things, enabling people to plan for the future while they are able.

By now she is incensed. If only, she thinks, Carl had seen Dr White sooner. She's a lovely person. Whenever they meet in the street, she always stops for a quick word. But she needs facts. She doesn't know what Carl actually told Dr Bromwich.

She's had Enduring Power of Attorney since 1995 on Dr White's recommendation.

She decides to ask for Carl's notes.

9

He'd got it wrong way round

The Practice Manager tells Ellie that they will both have to be interviewed by Carl's doctor who will decide whether it is in Carl's best interests for Ellie to see his notes. And that will only be with Carl's written permission. Ellie explains that she has had Power of Attorney for the past three years on Dr White's recommendation because Carl cannot manage his own affairs or even sign his own name. But the Practice Manager is adamant. Ellie, equally determined, fixes an appointment for a few days ahead.

She re-reads the open letter she'd asked Dr Bromwich for to get a reduction in her property rating:

> *...Mr Valente presented some four-and-a-half years ago with symptoms of depression which at that time were attributed to difficulties with his business...*

So, Ellie thinks, even after Dr White had diagnosed dementia Dr Bromwich still couldn't believe he'd got it wrong way round. The problems inside Carl's head had caused his business difficulties. That's why he went to the doctor. He'd become just as bad with jobs at home. That's why I went to the doctor.

They attend the interview with Dr Southam, taking with them a typewritten request for the notes. Beneath it is Carl's spidery scrawl stretching diagonally across most of the page with two letters legible. After a £50 payment, they receive a copy of his records going back to Carl's first visit to Dr Bromwich about his memory problems in August 1990.

By the time she has read the first page she is distraught.

10

'Carl, what do you want me to do about this?'

One word in Dr Bromwich's notes on Carl's first visit in August 1990 leaps out at Ellie: suicidal.

Suicidal.

My Carl's mental problems were so bad he was suicidal, she thinks. And I didn't understand how terrible he was feeling. The dafter he was, the angrier I got.

Oh, my poor Carl, I should have realised. What sort of wife have I been to you? And now it's too late to put things right.

Why didn't the doctor tell me?

At his two appointments that autumn he's feeling better and comes off the tablets. The next visit is a year later soon after Ellie had seen Dr Bromwich herself about Carl and come away believing the doctor would do something about it. But the record just says: TATT, a common medical term, which Ellie happens to know means 'tired all the time', and that Carl needs more time off.

So by the time in Carl's illness when other patients had been sent for specialist tests Dr Bromwich did nothing. If he had referred Carl to a specialist then, they would have closed the business before the debts mounted, she thinks again.

She's learned since joining the local Alzheimer's Society that Carl could have had a thyroid problem or a brain tumour. But all she's reading are Dr Bromwich's notes on Carl's poor memory and concentration yet doing nothing until he signs Carl off the sick. Then – only six days later – there's the note: '<u>UNFIT</u>' by the Head of Practice when she'd demanded a visit from him and he'd referred Carl to Dr White. She wonders if Dr Bromwich would ever have cottoned on.

Ellie phones the health authority's Complaints Manager and explains everything. She also complains about not being told that Carl was suicidal.

She receives a prompt reply from the Complaints Manager explaining that, although the complaint is out of time, she asked the current Head of Practice, Dr Corley, for his opinion. He said the doctors had always done their utmost to answer her concerns, and medical confidentiality prevented them from telling Ellie about Carl being suicidal. The letter ends by suggesting that if Ellie is dissatisfied she should see her solicitor.

Questions chase each other around inside Ellie's head. Is this a fob-off or is she pointing me in the right direction? Does any good come of seeing lawyers? Would I get Legal Aid? Do I have the stomach for a fight? I need all my energy to look after Carl.

But she remembers Carl's request: 'Nail the bastards!'

Straightaway an idea comes to mind and, wishing she'd thought of it before, she picks up the phone.

11

'Who cares for the carer?'

The phone rings. It's Ellie. I don't hear from her often. We're cousins and normally I hear about her through our mothers and see her only at weddings and funerals.

'Is that you, Renata? I hope I haven't caught you at a bad time,' she says.

I pick up the sadness in her voice. 'No! Don't worry,' I say, 'I'd nearly finished what I was doing.'

She tells me Carl's going downhill and I wouldn't recognise him now.

When they'd last dropped in they'd been flushed with the success of both businesses and the boys' academic achievements. Ellie had shown us the leaflet describing the themed guest rooms providing hospitality for guests from all over the world. She'd designed the interior herself and Carl had done all the DIY.

I'd realised something was amiss in the summer of 1994. I'd arranged to take my mother to Ellie's mother's funeral but when I phoned about the arrangements Carl seemed confused and uninformative. I'd shrugged it off at the time but there was a point, after the funeral, where both my mother and I had thought we'd overheard someone mention Carl and dementia.

'Oh, Ellie, I'm so sorry,' I say. 'I should have been in touch instead of relying on Mum to keep me up to date. It's a terrible illness and the carers feel the brunt of it. Sometimes people even accuse the wife or husband of causing it.'

'It's not that I'm ringing about,' Ellie says. 'It was three-and-a-half years before anyone told me what was wrong. And that was in a phone call from the consultant telling me to join the Alzheimer's Society.'

'Three-and-a-half years! How come?' I say.

I'm not a neurologist but I am a doctor who specialised in metabolic disorders (like cholesterol and diabetes) and also did some general practice. I do know that it's normally about a year, give or take a month or two. It can be difficult sometimes.

Ellie says that's what a local survey showed. But their GP had assumed that Carl's business problems were causing his illness when it was actually the other way round. If they'd known something was wrong with Carl sooner, the debts would have been nothing like £50,000. The business might even have been solvent. They could have sold or closed it, concentrated on the B&B, gone on cruises, taken holidays in the sun. The whole thing's been a nightmare.

It's a nightmare even when they *do* know what's wrong. I've had carers in tears over trying to cope. Many end up on anti-depressants and some in a psychiatric unit themselves. Amazing Ellie hasn't ended up the same way, I think. But she'd always coped with the hand life had dealt her and helped those in need. Someone you could depend on in times of trouble.

She says what upset her so much, though, was reading in Carl's medical records that he'd been suicidal and nobody had told her.

'What if I'd come home one day to find Carl had topped himself?' she says.

I ask her what she did about it.

'That's what I'm coming to,' she says. 'I spoke to the Complaints Manager and she wrote back with some guff about the complaint being out of time, medical confidentiality, the doctors always doing everything they could and if I didn't like it I should see my solicitor.'

No surprises there, I think.

Late diagnosis of dementia is far too common. Sometimes the patient or the carer is in denial. But too many health care workers see no point in early diagnosis. It'll manifest itself soon enough, you can't do anything about it and you can't have them leaning on the support services too soon. Never mind the individual's right to make his own decisions while he can, and to help with adapting gradually to the illness instead of being overwhelmed by a crisis.

But I can't comment without seeing the notes. I suggest that they come to lunch the next day when we'll both be around to go through everything and keep Carl entertained.

'I hoped you'd say that,' Ellie says. 'I feel better already. At least I'll know the truth.'

And the truth shall make you free. Or will it, I wonder.

12

'I'm going to pieces'

– Carl Valente

They drive over and although Carl appears to enjoy the occasion, his capacity for conversation is limited. He responds to each conversational overture with a pleasantry but cannot keep the interaction going.

After lunch, while Pete and Carl take the dog for a walk, Ellie and I start on the notes. Whatever failings this GP might have had, I think, poor record keeping and handwriting aren't among them. The entry for Carl's first visit reads:

> *Poor concentration/memory.* [These are known as
>   presenting symptoms]
> *Making mistakes in business.*
> *Lot of pressures: business, elderly mother* [just had second
>   stroke]*, dog died, property.*
> *Too busy + no holiday.*
> *Tense/irritable.*
> *Sleep OK but exhausted.*
> *Denies suicidal thoughts.*

I re-read it several times. It's unmistakably 'Denies suicidal thoughts'. *Denies.* Ellie must have misread it. The best reason anyone, medical or not, could have for not disclosing someone's suicidal thoughts to his next-of-kin is that he had none. Why, I wonder, did the Complaints Manager invoke the complex and irrelevant issue of medical confidentiality?

Somewhat perturbed, I leave comment until I've read all the notes. The rest of the entry for this consultation reads:

> *Drinking more than he should, recently up to 7–8 units/ day & admits it.*
> *Can stop if necessary.*
> *Discussion.*
> *Tape.* [relaxation tape]
> *Prothiaden* [anti-depressant] *75 mg at night. See 3/52.*

The GP requested a set of blood tests to check for alcohol damage, plus a routine cholesterol test. Depression, drinking too much or dementia could be causing Carl's intellectual (cognitive) difficulties. Prescribing a course of anti-depressants to see what effect they have on the cognitive difficulties is the recognised way of solving this familiar diagnostic conundrum in a patient with midlife stresses. If it's dementia there'll be little, if any, improvement in cognition; if it's depression, cognition should improve along with lightening of mood. But depression and dementia can co-exist. If the GP is still unsure after a few months he should refer the patient to a specialist.

I explain all this to Ellie and read the note for the follow-up visit:

> *Liver function tests normal.* [alcohol intake isn't affecting his liver]
> *Fasting fats borderline – advice re decrease fat intake.*
> *Beginning to feel better.*
> *Had a break + trying to work less hard.*

I'm side-tracked somewhat. The fasting fats, including cholesterol, aren't part of a first stage dementia screen. They have probably been measured as a routine. But having run a lipid clinic myself, I know that facile advice to cut down on fats is unlikely to have much effect especially if the patient isn't the cook. And Carl had probably forgotten about it by the time he got home.

Excess amounts of substances, e.g. cholesterol, in the bloodstream cause furring up of the blood vessels just as water pipes fur up in hard water areas. I'm suspecting that Carl has a vascular dementia, one of the causes being furred up arteries in the brain.

Carl's father had died of a heart attack aged fifty-six, his mother had had her first stroke before she was seventy, and Carl was a butcher whose wife was running a B&B serving full English breakfasts. A useful doctors' guide had been published in 1989 by two UK experts[3] defining borderline and ideal levels of cholesterol, and when to prescribe cholesterol lowering drugs. But I don't know the actual cholesterol value or how many other vascular risk factors, like raised blood pressure, Carl had.

But these are all things I'll come back to. Saying that I'll leave explanations about cholesterol for now, I tell Ellie that this is when things began to go wrong – *because Dr Bromwich didn't check on whether or not Carl's cognitive difficulties, his poor memory and concentration, which he saw the doctor about (the presenting symptoms) had improved on the anti-depressant.* Carl says he is *feeling* better. So that's all right then. Next patient, please.

The type of anti-depressant the GP chose can make some dementia patients' cognitive difficulties worse whilst they're on them even though their mood improves. It isn't necessarily a problem provided that you monitor both mood and cognitive function but the doctor hasn't done this.

I read the notes for the second follow-up visit in the autumn. Carl is feeling *much* better and can come off the anti-depressant – again with no check of his cognitive difficulties. It looks as if the doctor hasn't even thought of dementia.

In September 1991, Carl sees the GP again, complaining about being tired all the time, 'TATT'. It's a frequent complaint, hence the acronym. It has many causes including dementia, depression, other serious illnesses, boredom and overwork. The GP ascribes it to the latter:

> *Doing far too much + no holidays for 6/12. No physical*
> *symptoms.*
> *Discussion.*
> *Needs more time off.*

I wonder what had been happening during the past few months. Had the memory and concentration defects resolved, the truth being that Carl's dementia began much later? Was Carl's tax return fiasco a temporary aberration followed by dementia later?

If so, Ellie doesn't have a case. The doctors and the Complaints Manager dealt with the complaint adequately. The health authority's defence would be that this was a try-on to recover the lost £50,000 from the taxpayer.

'What do you think so far?' Ellie asks.

'I can't understand why Carl hasn't been back to the doctor between autumn 1990 and autumn 1991,' I say.

'But I went to see the doctor about Carl in March,' Ellie says.

She explains that it was because Carl was turning their B&B into Fawlty Towers at a time when he needed to reorganise his own business because of legislation[4] coming in that summer. She was worried that he wasn't up to it.

With good reason, I'm thinking. If this is a vascular dementia, it could have started in the part of the brain (called the executive cortex) dealing with planning and problem solving. In Alzheimer's dementia it normally starts in an area dealing with recent memory (called the hippocampus). But I'll explain more about that later.

Ellie says she came away from the doctor sure that he would see Carl and get him back to normal. She didn't want to interfere in Carl's business unnecessarily.

But her visit isn't recorded in Carl's notes. I can't understand it. In dementia the evidence of a close associate of the patient is vital.

'If the doctor really was taking your account seriously, he should have put it in Carl's notes as well, in case a different doctor saw him next time,' I say.

The period between Ellie's visit in March 1991 and Carl's in September 1991 is when Carl should have undergone detailed investigation. His illness was causing havoc. He could have had a brain tumour that needed aggressive treatment or a thyroid disorder which was readily treatable. It could have been done without breaching patient confidentiality if the GP had been monitoring the cognitive difficulties as he ought to have been.

I wonder if he's even recorded Ellie's visit in her own notes.

Time's going by so I start skim reading.

Carl starts another short course of the same anti-depressant when he sees the doctor about a year later. His business has closed by then and he now has symptoms of depression. From then on he consistently complains about poor concentration, still with no attempt by the GP to do something about it – apart from a visit when he is told to up the use of the relaxation tape to twice daily.

In spring 1993, there is an entry in different handwriting:

Concerned about poor concentration. Not overtly depressed.

Dr Bromwich's colleague, Dr Frankley, seeing Carl for the first time, orders a set of blood tests known as a dementia screen but doesn't mention his diagnosis to Carl at that stage. He wouldn't have wanted to alarm him without reason: further action would depend on the test results.

I tell Ellie about a case I'll always remember. I'd held a consultancy to a large chemical firm for some years and this fifty-odd-year-old manager's work performance had become so poor that he was facing redundancy. They wanted to make sure first that a medical problem wasn't the cause. The blood tests showed, somewhat to my surprise, that he had a thyroid problem and after treatment his work performance returned to normal.

Ellie says she's often wondered whether the dementia would have been picked up sooner if Carl had been an employee and been able to see a doctor at work. Quite possibly, I think.

Carl's blood tests were negative but, prompted by the other doctor's suspicions and Carl's complaint of 'going to pieces', Dr Bromwich referred him to a psychologist for formal tests.

Reading the lengthy referral letter, I'm gobsmacked.

'Why?' asks Ellie.

I must have spat the word out.

13

The right way round

Dr Bromwich's referral letter says as much about the doctor as the patient.

He describes Carl's progressive cognitive decline since 1990 as two distinct episodes of anxiety-depression followed by this third one in which it was noticed that Carl's performance was poor on a mental scoring test. He fails to mention Ellie's observations.

Unfortunately, the psychologist, about to go on long-term sick leave herself, failed to carry out the requested formal cognitive function tests, taking his word for it that making lists of things to remember was helpful enough. And she assessed Carl as not depressed.

'Did the psychologist contact you?' I ask.

'Contact me? No!' says Ellie.

I say that in cases like Carl's the observations of a close associate are vital. It's not rocket science – just common sense and correct clinical practice.

On his next visit Carl feels that further psychological input isn't needed and Dr Bromwich issues a RTW (Return to Work) note. I can see his dilemma.

The psychologist has excluded the depression diagnosis that Dr Bromwich was putting on Carl's sick notes – and remembering better by making lists isn't a clinical diagnosis. The GP, by requesting help from a diagnostic department, has been left without a diagnosis for Carl's sick note.

An RTW wasn't the GP's only option as I explain to Ellie:

The psychologist didn't do the formal tests she'd been asked to do. It's like we'd sent a reassuring report to the GP from the Path Lab without testing the blood sample because it looked all right in the sample tube. We just wouldn't do that, Ellie, I assure you. It's also rather like when we send out blood tests results that aren't what the doctor expected. When the doctor phones us – sometimes to complain we got the 'wrong' answer so he wants us to do the test again – it gets us talking to think of another way of finding out what's happening. We'd probably repeat the test on a fresh sample. Mistakes can happen even with the rigorous quality control we have in Path Labs. And maybe suggest other tests. The GP should have given Carl a sick note for two weeks instead of eight weeks and discussed it with the head of the psychology department.

The note by the Head of Practice, Dr Stratford, of his visit *six days later* states:

Did not understand the [several illegible words] *psychologist. Given clients at wife's B&B wrong meals/ wrong rooms. Confused. No concentration. Made hash of wife's books* [the B&B accounts]. *UNFIT. 8/52* [sick note for eight weeks]

His terse handwritten referral letter to the dementia specialist reads:

This man has been seen by the psychologist because of loss of memory, so bad that he had to give up his business [he's got it the right way round]. *He now 'helps' his wife – but this is more of a hindrance. He forgets what he has done & gets it all wrong. He wired an electrical plug the wrong way*

— luckily it was discovered in time. His wife wonders about early Alzheimer's. He seems very unconcerned & thinks it will all get better.

Thanks to Ellie, the Return to Work note brought matters to a head.

I think again of how she coped for three years without knowing what was wrong, paying off the massive debts, and running their home and the B&B with Carl's hindrance. I'm not surprised, though. Her goodness and strength come from her poor but loving childhood home and her absolute Christian faith.

She says she often wonders what they'd have made of Carl at the Job Centre. We recall an eighties sitcom that pitted dispirited jobseekers against disillusioned Job Centre staff. But it isn't funny. Carl would have been a dangerous liability in any workplace by then.

'It feels,' I say, 'like you hired a taxi when you weren't sure of the way. The driver, refusing to listen when you said you thought he'd taken a wrong turning, drove miles up a narrow track with grass growing down the middle until you ended up in a farmyard full of barking dogs.'

Seeing Pete and Carl coming back, she says they'll have to leave soon. She's expecting new arrivals at the B&B. I tell her: 'Ellie, I can put your mind at rest on one thing. Carl was not suicidal. He *denies* suicidal thoughts. Look!'

She reads it. Her face clears then she frowns. She seems lost in thought for a minute. Then she turns to me and says: 'But why didn't...?'

I know what she's thinking.

14

'The wounds I might have healed
The sorrow and the smart
But evil is wrought by want of thought
As well as want of heart'
— Thomas Hood, 1799–1845

Next morning I wake up pondering on why the Complaints Manager didn't explain that Carl *denied* suicidal thoughts but I decide to finish reading the GP records first.

I start on Dr Bromwich's open letter which Ellie needed for the ratings department:

December 1994

TO WHOM IT MAY CONCERN

Mr Valente presented some 4½ years ago with symptoms of depression which at the time were attributed to difficulties within his personal business.

There were no symptoms specific to depression and, worse, Dr Bromwich has released his disastrous wrong assumption from the confines of Carl's confidential medical notes to a public department. The letter continues:

He was treated for a short time with counselling and anti-depressants and appeared to improve. However, about

2½ years ago there was a recurrence of symptoms and in particular, it was noticed that he had considerable problems with concentration and memory and he was referred to the local psychiatrist. A subsequent CT scan of the brain and EEG showed mild atrophy which was felt to account for his symptoms.

Carl may have *felt* better but the *cognitive* difficulties, which Dr Bromwich had ignored for nearly three years despite Carl and Ellie's frequent complaints to him, were constant and worsening. It was Dr Bromwich's colleague, Dr Frankley, who, on seeing Carl for the first time, suspected the diagnosis which the local dementia specialist (a psychiatrist in this health authority: in others it can be a neurologist) confirmed on Carl's first visit to her. *The main purpose of the CT scan was to exclude a brain tumour.* And *the diagnosis is primarily clinical* because evidence of cerebral atrophy (brain shrinkage) on CT, or even the more sensitive MRI scan, is not necessarily present in early dementia.

The letter continues:

Mrs Valente presented some 3½ years ago with symptoms of anxiety, mainly related to concern about her husband's physical and mental health, a year ago became quite severely depressed and has taken anti-depressants intermittently since. Her mental state appears relatively stable but she feels a need to reduce her commitment to work.

Dr Bromwich's own notes show that her concern was *entirely* over her husband's *mental* health. Most carers need some psychiatric support as the dementia progresses – even without a debt mountain. This paragraph would have been better phrased thus: 'Now that Mrs Valente has paid off the debts she wishes to be free to devote more time to her husband's increasing needs by reducing her work load'.

Ellie asked Dr Bromwich for his opinion on Carl's mental

state, not her own, yet he has released his regrettable assessment of her from the confines of her confidential medical records to the same public department.

I feel outraged. Readers of this open letter could easily gain the wrong impression of them both. Ellie's had wind of rumours from time to time. It's a small enough town for news to spread of someone's encounters with creditors, the DSS and the ratings department – and of long-term sick notes for psychiatric problems culminating in a disputed Return to Work note with the gossips adding their ha'p'orth. Professional confidentiality isn't one hundred per cent reliable especially when the source is a doctor's misleading open letter intended for a public department.

The notes on Carl's 1995 formal psychological tests showing that he was unfit to drive beg the question of what they would have shown when Ellie expressed concerns about his driving to the doctors. I think of all the cases I have heard of where families have taken matters into their own hands when faced with the authorities' indolence or disbelief. One mechanically minded relative felt impelled to surreptitiously remove the distributor arm from the engine of an unfamiliar car in an unlit garage in order to stop the person driving (a tricky solution that solved the problem but is inapplicable to most modern cars).

I read the notes on Carl's sad experience after the Galanthamine trial ended. Ellie's handwritten request to Dr Southam, Dr Bromwich's successor, enclosing a copy of the newspaper article on Aricept[5] reads:

> *There is another drug already licensed and available on the NHS. Could Carl go on this ASAP? Thank you for all your help in a very difficult situation.*

Dr Southam's note on Ellie's follow-up phone call whilst Dr White is doing her best to get hold of the substitute Aricept for Carl states:

Wife very distressed. Prepared to fund it herself.

Fortunately, Carl's consultant was able after a struggle to obtain the Aricept for Carl on a named patient basis and he improved again.

I've reached the day when Ellie accesses Carl's notes. Even reading them has left me feeling drained. I'll think about the Complaints Manager's letter tomorrow. Ellie never had that option. I'm off out shopping this afternoon where Ellie's fear and loneliness hit me hard.

Bereft

*In a shopping complex
come sounds from a grand piano
lacking meaning and melody,
psychotic, surreal.*

*These keys move of their own volition
no pianist needed. She's in a suspense film.
She shudders, alone
on a long walkway like a sealed tube –
except for the statues
standing aside, staring at space.*

*Instant logic prevails:
the piano is playing
computer concoctions.*

*Her friend's husband keeps failing to light
the gas cooker. He can't be left
by himself. She's frightened, alone
in their home that's like a sealed tube –
outside are the doctors
standing aside, staring at space.*

There's a diagnosis when four years on
her husband can't find
the cooker. He has dementia.

He's a piano bereft
of a pianist's touch.

15

'I am playing the right notes'

– Eric Morecambe, comedian

Next morning I read the Complaints Manager's letter which begins:

> *Thank you for contacting the health authority recently to advise us of your concerns following the care and treatment provided to your husband, Mr Carl Valente, by Dr Bromwich (deceased). As we discussed, the NHS Complaints Procedure introduced in April 1996[6] has timescales associated with the original incident being complained about i.e. within 12 months.*
>
> *The first stage of the procedure also requires the relevant general practitioner to respond to a complaint. The whole procedure is based around trying to resolve a complaint by conciliatory means and is in no way disciplinary nor is there any financial recompense by way of compensation for perceived grievances.*
>
> *Although I do not have any written information, from the verbal history you provided over the telephone it would seem that you feel your husband should have been diagnosed with Alzheimer's disease before the actual date in 1994. As your husband had been visiting the doctor since 1990/1991 with symptoms being associated with stress and anxiety I understand*

that you feel his doctor should have made a diagnosis earlier.
You feel this would then have enabled you to make earlier
decisions about the future of your business ventures to avoid
the financial situation you found yourself in.

Given Ellie's capacity for plain speaking, this feels like either an
attempt to square the circle or a failure to grasp Ellie's complaint:
Carl's symptoms from August 1990 onwards were of dementia and
had Dr Bromwich referred him to a specialist when he should have
done, between spring and autumn 1991, they could have closed the
business whilst it was solvent.

The phrase 'your business ventures' grates:

1. A business venture is a speculative undertaking involving some degree of risk. Carl and Ellie were running
   successful established businesses.
2. Legislation, not speculation, forced Carl to make a business decision to downsize which was beyond him due to
   undiagnosed cognitive impairment.
3. The sole relevance of Ellie's B&B business is that it
   cleared the debts, preventing bankruptcy with the loss
   of their home and livelihood – and premature depend-
   ency on state support services.

If only I'd known sooner about the dementia, Ellie said yesterday.
If only I'd known sooner about the symptoms, I think, I'd have
told them to get a specialist's opinion quick even if it meant paying
for it. Something had been seriously amiss inside Carl's head for
around a year by the time Dr Bromwich should have referred him.
It may not have been possible to make the diagnosis then – *but
dementia could not have been excluded.* They'd have kept Carl
under close review.

And the most optimistic answer in summer 1991 to the
question of whether Carl was likely to get better soon would have

been: 'I wouldn't bank on it'. On that basis, the common sense decision would have been to sell Carl's business.

The next two paragraphs of the letter are:

> *I have spoken to Dr Corley* [the current Head of Practice] *and he has confirmed that during the last few years the practice have tried to respond to your concerns. Unfortunately the practice do not feel that there is anything further they can do to resolve those concerns. He is aware that Dr Bromwich (before his demise) and Dr Stratford the then Head of Practice (prior to retirement) had discussed your concerns with you. At the time they had indicated that they had done everything they could to identify the cause of the symptoms and did make appropriate referrals which resulted in a diagnosis.*
>
> *The doctors regret your ongoing distress but feel that they can add nothing further as the doctors involved did take appropriate actions.*

Dr Corley was right: the doctors made the appropriate referrals and took the appropriate actions. But at the wrong time. Like Eric Morecambe grabbed André Previn by the lapels and said he was playing the right notes. But in the wrong order.

This was not a comedy show: it was a real life nightmare for a sick man and his lonely, bewildered and exhausted wife.

The next paragraph reads:

> *You referred to an entry in your husband's notes about "suicidal" thoughts. This would not be divulged without his express permission. This again, is part of the doctor/ patient relationship which requires complete patient confidentiality.*

This is the 'Denies suicidal thoughts' note that Ellie had misread and been devastated by. Why, I wonder, wasn't Ellie given the same crumb of comforting truth that I had given her yesterday, perhaps in a sentence like this: 'Dr Corley suggests you carefully re-read the first page of your husband's notes where it is clearly stated that he *denies* suicidal thoughts.'

The most likely explanation is that Dr Corley, with a broad picture of the case and a lot on his mind as Head of Practice, accepted Ellie's misreading of the suicidal ideation note without referring to Carl's records and told the Complaints Manager that medical confidentiality would preclude divulging such information. The letter concludes:

> *In view of the comments from Dr Corley and the length of time which has elapsed since 1994, I must confirm that the NHS Complaints Procedure cannot be invoked in your case.*
>
> *I appreciate that this will distress you but I can only suggest that if you wish to take things further you should instruct your solicitor.*

You should instruct your solicitor. But the complaint was not a belated try-on: 'Hey, Ellie, that happened to somebody I got talking to in the pub and he got a hundred grand out of them.' It was late because it was only in 1998 that Ellie had good evidence from the local dementia survey that the diagnostic delay was excessive.

I check the guidance notes on the NHS complaints procedures:[6]

> *4.11…There is discretion to extend this time limit where it would be unreasonable in the circumstances of a particular case for the complaint to have been made earlier and where it is still possible to investigate the facts of the case…*
> *4.12…The discretion to vary the time limit should be used flexibly and sensitively.*

> *4.13 When a complaint is made outside the time limit,*
> *it will be for the complaints manager, or appropriate*
> *family health services practitioner, to take responsibility for*
> *considering an extension of the time limit.*
> *4.14 If the discretionary extension of the time limit is*
> *rejected by the complaints manager, then the procedure*
> *will be...*[list of complainant's options follows from
> resolution at local level to the NHS Ombudsman].

Irrespective of why the Complaints Manager exercised her
discretion not to extend the time limit, she had a duty to inform
Ellie of her options for continuing to pursue the matter through
the NHS complaints procedures.

The guidance includes this:

> *Wherever possible the complainant's concerns should be*
> *addressed constructively, while remaining scrupulously fair*
> *to staff.*

and this:

> *A hostile, or defensive, reaction to the complaint is more*
> *likely to encourage the complainant to seek information*
> *and a remedy through the courts. In the early part of the*
> *process, it may not be clear whether the complainant simply*
> *wants an explanation and an apology, with an assurance*
> *that any failures in service will be rectified for the future,*
> *or whether the complainant is in fact seeking information*
> *with formal litigation in mind.*

With £50,000 involved, the Complaints Manager may have
concluded that litigation was what Ellie had in mind. But that
begs the question posed by Margaret Brazier in *Medicine, Patients*

and the Law[7] of whether having litigation in mind when seeking answers constitutes misuse of the complaints procedure. Fairness is what concerns people.

Delayed investigation of impaired cognitive function can result in denial of these rights:

- To make your own decisions while you are able
- To treatment in the early stages when it is most likely to help
- To protection from injury at the hands of the carer whose patience snaps
- Of the carer to help and support
- Of the innocent to protection from the predations or violence of those whom dementia has disinhibited
- Of road users to protection from those whom dementia has rendered unfit to drive.

I make some notes on dementia for Ellie before we decide what to do.

Years later I shall discover that the solicitors' Legal Aid extension application contained the erroneous declaration that Ellie had not sought an alternative method of dispute resolution prior to litigation – although when the complainant has done so details including outcome and a copy of the correspondence are required with the application form. When I reminded the solicitors of this I was told that it was irrelevant.

PART 2

On Dementia

'Of all the things I've lost,
I miss my mind the most.'

– Mark Twain

16

'Listen to the patient, he's telling you the diagnosis'
– William Osler, 1849–1919

This is as true now as ever it was. Objective investigations like the doctor's examination findings, blood tests, biopsies, X-rays, and scans have their limitations too. You can miss as much, at greater expense and inconvenience, by not taking a good history as you can by not ordering enough tests or by not assessing them correctly.

By the end of the first consultation, the doctor should have a mental list of possible reasons for the patient's complaint: the differential diagnosis. At the other extreme is the definitive diagnosis: what the doctor knows for certain is the problem. It might, as with some skin diseases, be within a minute or two of seeing the patient: the so-called 'spot' (i.e. on-the-spot) diagnosis – satisfying for both patient and doctor if it's (a) easy to treat (b) rare. It's like a *Diagnostics Road Show*: the patient comes in with something rare; the doctor, who's only seen one case before when he was a student, cleverly recognises it; the patient goes home the proud owner of a rare disease. If some top specialists hadn't a clue what it was, that's even better.

Definitive diagnosis may come only after further investigation of varying duration and complexity, the ultimate being at post-mortem. Somewhere between these extremes lies presumptive diagnosis. It's what the doctor thinks is most likely, usually after ruling out other conditions from the original differential diagnosis list by means of definitive tests for specific causes, such as thyroid disorders. These are known as exclusion diagnoses. But, because *dementia is not an exclusion diagnosis*[8] i.e. it cannot be ruled out, it must remain on the list of possibles, the differential diagnosis. Management and treatment before the diagnosis declares itself one way or another is based on a presumptive diagnosis. In other words, diagnosis is not an 'Is the door open or is it shut?' question.

Improving the certainty of a presumptive (most likely – but still bearing other possibilities in mind) diagnosis or making a definitive diagnosis may need referral to a specialist – and, crucially, the passage of enough time for the disease to declare itself during which the doctor must help the patient to manage the problem. As a rough guide, GPs work on probabilities, based partly on symptoms and partly on the frequency of the condition; hospital specialists investigate possibilities. One of the great skills of general practice is judging when to refer to a specialist.

Dementia diagnosis

As we saw in Chapters 14 and 15, Carl had no symptoms specific to depression, his presenting complaints being entirely of poor intellectual function. So, out of the three main diagnoses (depression, drinking too much alcohol and dementia), dementia was the most likely.[9] And the silly mistakes he was making were suggestive of dementia rather than depression where the mistakes tend to be of omission (procrastinating and not completing tasks).

But severe stress and depression in a middle-aged man are far commoner than early-onset dementia. The GP's decision to try him on an anti-depressant and advise him to cut down on alcohol was reasonable at first.

Carl attended for two follow-up appointments that autumn, the GP established that he was feeling better, the liver function tests were normal and he had stopped drinking. But that was it. The question 'How are your memory and concentration?' doesn't seem to have occurred to Dr Bromwich.

Ellie's first visit to him in March 1991, complaining that Carl's mistakes, so unlike him, were affecting both businesses and their marriage resulted only in tranquillisers and a relaxation tape – for her. He didn't act on his stated intention to 'See husband', simply telling Carl he was doing too much when he happened to turn up soon after.

In very old people, some cognitive impairment may be disregarded as ageing with the risk: benefit ratio of treatment making its usefulness questionable. But cognitive impairment in younger patients with huge impact on them and their families demands full investigation and intensive management.

Fully treatable causes e.g. thyroid disorders are easily excluded. The big breakthrough came in the second half of the last century with fast accurate blood tests of thyroid function. Nowadays, they are part of a dementia screen (provided the doctor thinks of the possibility) and even your cat can have its thyroid function tests done by the local vet (albeit for an irregular pulse rather than cognitive decline).

Brain scans detect conditions presenting as dementia that need aggressive treatment (e.g. brain tumours). That is their main use in the early stages when they may not pick up brain shrinkage caused by brain cell destruction (cerebral atrophy).

Similarly, psychometric tests might simply confirm the cognitive impairment or indicate functional causes, e.g. psychiatric or severe stress, or be consistent with dementia and even its type. Importantly, they may also show up disproportionate deficits in specific areas of brain function that could affect driving e.g. visuo-spatial impairment, poor judgement or slow responses.

The difficulty for the clinician, though, is that some patients with cognitive defects will develop dementia and some won't.[10] Some patients do recover completely even from serious cognitive impairment if severe stressors and/or depressive responses can be dealt with. The consequences of sticking a wrong label like dementia on a patient can be as devastating as failing to suspect it.

Whatever the tests show, the person must be kept under

careful review until the problem declares itself. Conditions like high blood pressure, diabetes and raised cholesterol and other blood fats, collectively known as lipids, which may slow the progress of the dementia and prevent further dementia caused by strokes, should be dealt with anyway. It's good medical practice.

By the second half of the last century, lipid profiles, like thyroid function tests, were readily measured in general hospital Path Labs. Cholesterol, for example, can clog up arteries just as pipes get furred up in hard water areas, as we shall see in Chapter 17, restricting the supply of oxygen and nutrients in the blood to the brain. And we know that Carl's cholesterol was somewhat raised, his father died young of a heart attack and his mother from a series of strokes.

If your car develops a fault in the engine management system, the local mechanic will check the battery, contacts and plugs, maybe run some screening tests or get the main agent to take a look. Even they may not be any the wiser, given the complexity of these systems, until the problem declares itself or is revealed by further diagnostic tests. Meanwhile you would use your judgement, based on their expert advice, on whether to risk driving your car through the centre of Birmingham, around Spaghetti Junction or up the M6 on a Friday evening. Similarly, Carl and Ellie, had they received timely expert advice would have used their judgement and closed Carl's business.

I imagine what would have happened if Carl had received specialist advice instead of them both getting a relaxation tape off the GP. He'd have closed his business with a sigh of relief in 1991, and they'd have enjoyed life-enhancing Mediterranean fare in their sunny garden knowing they were doing all they could in the light of modern knowledge to snatch whatever moments of happiness remained for them.

17

Plumbers v electricians

The human body is like a house. The heart pumps blood containing oxygen and nutrients through blood vessels (arteries) to all parts of the body like the pump sends hot water from the boiler through pipes to heat all the rooms in a house. The heart must work against gravity to send blood up to the brain like hot water being pumped to the radiators in an upstairs office.

Plumbing: heart, blood vessels, strokes and vascular dementia
Put simply, blood vessels can become narrowed or completely blocked in a process called atheroma, equivalent to pipes furring up in hard water areas. Anitschow found back in 1913 that the furring up was by patchy cholesterol-rich deposits called plaques and 'confidently stated that there can be no atheroma without cholesterol, neatly upstaging all subsequent work in the area' – as Professor Paul Durrington equally neatly puts it in the introduction to his textbook, *Hyperlipidaemia: Diagnosis and Management.*[11]

When your cholesterol is too high plaque forms on the walls of the larger arteries causing blood clotting on the surface which can block the artery completely. When your blood isn't runny enough for other reasons blood clotting, thrombosis, can happen in the smaller arteries in the brain where the blood flow against gravity can be sluggish. When a piece of blood clot in a larger artery elsewhere in the body breaks off, called an embolus, it may get stuck in one of these small arteries. It's like circulating gunge in the central heating system blocking up smaller pipes.

The heart is a muscle so it needs its own blood supply. That comes via the heart's own (coronary) arteries. If one of them gets blocked completely the area of heart muscle it supplies dies through lack of oxygen: a myocardial infarct, a.k.a. heart attack or 'coronary'. A partial blockage may only cause trouble during exercise when the heart is working harder causing heart muscle pain – angina.

The brain too needs oxygen and nutrients to do its work. Its blood supply is via the carotid arteries in the neck at each side of the windpipe, and the basilar artery at the back of the neck. If the blood supply to an area of the brain is cut off by blockages either in these arteries or their smaller branches, the brain cells they supply are damaged or destroyed. This is what happens in a stroke.

How big the blocked artery is and where it is in the brain determines what symptoms you get and which side of the body is affected. If not immediately fatal, the blockage can mean anything from paralysis down one side of the body with speech problems and a long convalescence to a transient ischaemic attack (TIA) or a mini-stroke that's over in minutes or a day if the artery is very small.

A blockage formed on the arterial wall itself is a thrombotic stroke. A piece of plaque breaking off a larger artery to become stuck in a smaller artery (arteriole) in the brain causes an embolic stroke. One culprit is too much 'bad' LDL cholesterol in the blood stream encouraging plaque formation.

This can be offset to some extent if you have enough 'good' HDL-cholesterol in your blood: it's an indicator of how well your arteries are being cleared of cholesterol. It's having the right balance between good and bad cholesterol that counts because all cells in the body, especially the brain, need some cholesterol. The ratio between good and bad cholesterol is a useful guide to your risk of artery blockage.

In these conditions the blood may become too thick to circulate through the many small arteries in the brain:

- Raised blood levels of a fat called triglyceride as can happen in overweight and Type 2 diabetes
- Tiny blood cells called platelets which help the blood to clot after a wound becoming too sticky (platelet aggregation)
- Raised levels of various other blood clotting factors causing clots (thrombi) to form on the arterial wall especially at the site of a plaque.

The other type of stroke (haemorrhagic) happens when high blood pressure causes bleeding through the arterial walls into the brain. It's particularly likely to happen if the heart has to work harder forcing the blood at high pressure through arteries whose walls are thickened and weakened by plaque. Someone with high blood pressure plus raised blood fats and/or blood that's too thick, i.e. has a combination of what are known as vascular risk factors, is at risk of having a stroke of some sort. And somebody with only borderline abnormalities of each may be more at risk than somebody with, say, a higher cholesterol but no other risk factors.

Fisher, in 1968, laid the foundations of the vascular dementia concept by postulating that significant mental impairment was usually the result of strokes in the thinking part of the brain.[12] A large brain artery can become blocked destroying enough brain tissue for sudden onset of dementia and the other features of a stroke. Or over time, a number of very small arteries become blocked damaging only a small area of the brain at a time until sufficient brain cells are destroyed to affect thinking: this is known as multi-infarct dementia.

Electrics: the brain, the nervous system and what happens to the brain cells in dementia

The human brain weighs just over three pounds (about 1.5 kilograms) much less than muscles but thinking needs a surprising amount of oxygen and nutrients, whether you're an astro-physicist or a couch potato.

It consists of:

1. Cerebral cortex (grey matter, thinking part) divided into a right and a left hemisphere and sub-divided into:
   (a) frontal lobes (at the front, behind the forehead) containing the executive cortex dealing with problems, planning and decision making
   (b) parietal lobes (at the sides) dealing with sensory input; temporal lobes dealing with language (at the sides)
   (c) occipital lobes (at the back) dealing with everything visual, including reading
   (d) limbic system (deep inside the brain) dealing with learning and memory
2. Cerebellum dealing with movement and balance
3. Brain stem (oldest part of the brain) dealing with automatic primitive functions like breathing, heartbeat, etc.

Millions of cells make up the brain. The cell bodies together form the grey matter. They have long projections, 'micro-wires', called axons grouped in bundles forming the white matter.

The brain functions through tiny electric currents passing from the cell body down the axons like messages down telephone wires and across the gap to the receiver (called a receptor) on the next cell. Then on to the next cell and so on until thought has been translated into action whether that's reading, speaking, running or problem solving.

The parts of the brain dealing with automatic functions like breathing take their cue from physical and chemical signals. For example, there is a sensor, the respiratory centre, in the primitive part of the brain. When carbon dioxide builds up to a certain level in the blood (normally when the levels of oxygen in the body are getting low) messages in the form of tiny electric currents go down nerves from the respiratory centre to the muscles that expand and contract the chest. You breathe in and out taking in oxygen and breathing out carbon dioxide.

The electric currents are transmitted across the gap (called a synapse) between brain cells by several different substances, called neurotransmitters. In dementia, the damaged brain cells are short of the thinking brain's transmitter substance, acetylcholine, so the current can't get across the gap between affected cells. In vascular dementia the first part of the brain to be affected tends to be that dealing with planning, problem solving and abstract reasoning. Skills needed to run a business for years and provide figures for your tax returns. In Alzheimer's disease the first area of the brain to be affected is the hippocampus, part of the limbic system, dealing with recent memory. That's why people with Alzheimer's disease can't remember what they've just had for lunch but might be able to tell you what they had at their wedding reception.

The rationale of the mainstream drug treatments of dementia is to ensure that any acetylcholine which the brain cells can produce is conserved to keep the connections between the brain cells working for as long as possible. They don't target the initial damage to the cells that causes the lack of acteylcholine.

Once the brain cells become unable to produce any acetylcholine at all the drug stops working. Dementia, whether it starts as Alzheimer's, vascular or both, then picks off other areas of the brain until it reaches its final destination: the primitive part controlling basic bodily functions.

What causes the damage in the first place?
For a long time the answer rather depended on which side of the Atlantic you lived. This is where a popular science article by Will

Block in lifeenhancement.com[13] (well worth a read) and a survey of the literature (if you can face it) come in.

In Europe it was the 'electricians' who prevailed: neurologists, academic types who study brain biophysics and biochemistry, just as Alzheimer and his colleagues studied its microscopy a century ago. The problem's inside the brain cells: it's an innate, even genetic, degenerative disorder, something even the neurologists are only now beginning to probe. That's neurology for you.

In America and Canada from the 1970s onwards, the 'plumbers', vascular specialists, concentrated on fixing things in their department: furred up heart and carotid arteries, high blood pressure, diabetes, obesity, high blood fat levels, etc. They were spurred on, ironically, by the calls to action from a neurologist originally from this side of the Atlantic, Professor Vladimir Hachinsky, in the British journal *The Lancet* in 1974 and again in 1992.[14,15]

Hachinsky's family had escaped to Canada from Stalinist Russia when he was a teenager and his thirty-three-year-old mother suffered a stroke from which, fortunately, she recovered. It could have been what drove him to become a Professor of Neurology, disproving his early self-rating as 'not smart enough to become a neurologist'.

In his 1992 *Lancet* review with the provocative title: *Preventable senility: a call for action against the vascular dementias* he recognised three stages of dementia: brain at risk, pre-dementia, and established dementia. At Stages 1 and 2, management of vascular risk factors: high blood pressure, smoking, diabetes, hyperlipidaemia (cholesterol and triglycerides), and obesity can slow the cognitive decline. By Stage 3 optimising the limited brain cell function becomes the mainstay of treatment. In 1990–1991 a specialist would probably have assessed Carl as being at Stage 1, the 'brain at risk' stage based on his cognitive difficulties and evidence of vascular risk factors.

Summarising how treatment of vascular risk factors looked to specialists by September 1991, vascular dementia is remediable to an extent that depends on the particular risk factor(s) concerned and how far advanced the condition is. By managing the vascular risk factors you can at least minimise the risk of further damage to the brain cells.

By then many consultants in my speciality were, like me, running lipid (blood fat) clinics. We were in a good position to refer Hachinski's Stage 1 or 2 cases to neurologists or specialists in vascular disorders to begin treatment as soon as possible both on behalf of the patients themselves and to quantify for the benefit of others the effect, if any, of *timely* (the sooner the better) vascular risk factor modification.

When seeing a case like Carl in my lipid clinic, that's what I'd have done. I liked the family cook to attend to ensure they understood the practicalities of the diet. It's unlikely that a worried close relative accompanying the patient wouldn't have availed herself of the opportunity to tell her side of the story. But you can't put the clock back.

We would discover later from Carl's full records that his formal diagnosis was atherosclerotic, a type of vascular, dementia with borderline increases in three vascular risk factors and a positive family history of cardio- and cerebro-vascular disease. By the time he was diagnosed he'd reached Hachinski's Stage 3 when treatment becomes centred on optimising the limited brain function but as we saw earlier Ellie had a struggle to obtain even this.

Encouragement for the plumbers had come in the late 1980s. Statins, the best-ever cholesterol lowering drugs, and other treatments became widely available, facilitating acceptance of the link between raised cholesterol and heart attacks. The focus switched to research on the relative contributions of vascular risk factors, including cholesterol, to strokes and dementia.

Although it feels like a more fundamental approach, progress felt like two steps forward, one step back – or the reverse. Running through the rock of essential scientific scepticism was a seam of die-hard incredulity persisting today in the form of The International Network of Cholesterol Skeptics.[16] Bhatnagar and Durrington's 1989 guidelines on managing borderline cholesterol levels to reduce the risk of a heart attack[17] begin with this 1972 quote of medical writer Dr Richard Asher's:

> *Please do not write any more articles about cholesterol and coronary disease and the diet and drugs which are supposed to influence them. The facts about coronary disease are these: the less atheromatous your ancestors, the harder your water, and the more habitual exercise you take, the less likely you are to be troubled by it. Do stop bothering about whether your fats are saturated or unsaturated, help yourselves liberally to butter and stop propagating these erroneous legends.*

concluding:

> *This remains too frequently the view of medical practitioners in Britain…prescience had on this rare occasion deserted Dr Asher.*

If dementia is an innately determined degenerative condition, is scepticism about the value of treating vascular risk factors, including cholesterol, the voice of reason – or the voice of a latter-day Richard Asher whose prescience has deserted him?

18

'Theories have four stages of acceptance:
(i) this is worthless nonsense
(ii) this is an interesting, but perverse, point of view
(iii) this is true but quite unimportant
(iv) I always said so.'
– JBS Haldane, 1963, *The Journal of Genetics*

As we saw in the last chapter, by the early 1990s, mainstream medical opinion on the link between cholesterol and heart attacks had progressed from stage (i) to stage (iv). The equivalent event in the thinking part of the brain, a stroke or series of strokes maybe culminating in dementia, had received less attention.

At that time, I was aware of the accumulating evidence that control of vascular risk factors, like high blood pressure, Type 2 diabetes, and raised blood fats: 'bad' LDL cholesterol and triglyceride, might prevent and even slow the progress of dementia including the Alzheimer type.[18,19,20,21,22] In ageing populations chronic degenerative conditions like dementia were robbing too many sufferers and their carers of a happy retirement – and placing an enormous financial burden on their country's health and social services. Something had to be done[18] and, during the nineteen-nineties, it became an area of 'intense international research interest'.[23]

By the turn of the New Millennium the evidence had mounted. Expert reviews of the importance of vascular risk factor management in dementia had appeared for clinicians in specialist and mainstream journals worldwide including the UK [23,24,25,26] and one handbook for non-specialist clinicians.[27] In summary, vascular risk factors played a part in both vascular and Alzheimer type dementia with some evidence that their treatment might slow the decline.

But Sod's Law of Biology Evidence works like Newton's Third Law of Motion: for every result there is an equal and opposite result. Biology abounds with paradox and confounding factors, known and unknown.

Twin studies are a good example. Some identical twin pairs unequivocally discordant (one twin gets the condition but the other doesn't) for dementia in early case reports[28,29,30] were found when DNA testing became available to be non-identical. The researchers hadn't done the experiment they thought they were doing (showing whether there was an environmental as well as genetic factor at work) so their conclusion was wrong. The simple explanation for the discordance rate between these supposedly identical (monozygotic) twins was they were genetically different (fraternal/dizygotic) twins who happened to look the same. Right?

Well, no. The Swedish HARMONY study of DNA-proved identical twins showed that there were also environmental factors at work.[31] And a study using the Norwegian Twin Register showed that heredity was the major causal factor in Alzheimer's disease whereas environmental factors dominate in vascular dementia.[32] That being so, the condition could either be prevented or its progress slowed to an extent depending on how soon it was identified and the strength of the genetic effect.

Where the cause is *entirely* genetic (called deterministic), like Huntington's disease, (very early rapidly progressive dementia with involuntary movements), there is no treatment and no cure: genetic counselling and support are the only options. But these account for only 5% of the genetic causes. The vast majority are risk genes: like the genetic variant of Apolipoprotein E (linked to cholesterol metabolism) they definitely increase the risk *but not the certainty* of developing Alzheimer type dementia.[33]

It's not a question of: 'Is the door open (curable with, say, thyroid hormone) or is it shut (incurable as in Huntington's disease)?' The door is ajar: manageable by correcting other risk factors.

The gold standard for evaluating treatment is the large, well conducted, randomised placebo-controlled trial. It comes as no surprise that results are still awaited for the efficacy of treating vascular risk factors in dementia.

The difficulties are enormous: practical, financial, and ethical. Among the practical problems are the various types of vascular dementia and their different risk factors, the ways of managing them, and the different ways of measuring cognition each with its own advocates. One study might show a difference between treated and untreated groups whereas another study doesn't, simply because the two studies' criteria for defining the dementia sub-type were different.

The practical problems of seeing a trial through to satisfactory completion enhance the difficulty of getting and maintaining research funding. No wonder there's a saying that the only way to convince a funding committee they won't be wasting their money on your trial is to show them the one you made earlier.

Carl's experience in the Galanthamine trial is sad testimony to some of the ethical difficulties. He responded very well but his luck ran out when the trial ended – and with it the supply of Galanthamine before it could be licensed for use in this country.

I reflect on the anecdotal evidence of primary prevention (not letting a disease get started) that's been known for many years. Many chain-smoking (single vascular risk factor) inhabitants of hill villages on Greek islands live to a ripe (well, wizened) old age, seemingly untroubled by the heart attacks, strokes and dementia that afflict the elderly in northwest Europe who so often have combinations of vascular risk factors.

The impression had been around for a while that dementia rates in European countries seem to pattern those of heart attacks: a high to low gradient from the north west to the south east. This has been linked to diet: NW Europe – high dairy produce and fatty meats with low fruit and veg intake; SE Europe – fish, sunflower and olive oil with high fruit and veg intake.[34,35,36]

At the other geographical and medical extreme are patients whose dementia is so advanced that tertiary prevention (stopping established disease getting worse) would be useless. So what's needed is secondary prevention: avoidance or alleviation of a condition by detection and appropriate management either before symptoms appear (by screening tests) or as soon after that as possible. This means management of the vascular risk factors before or during the 'brain at risk' stage. Vascular risk factors are what they say they are: factors that increase the risk of some form of vascular disease including dementia and strokes with dementia. They aren't the cause of dementia in the same way as bacteria and viruses cause infections; they are more akin to how an illness or injury that causes immobility increases susceptibility to infection.

Raised cholesterol is an example worth looking at again.

To dispel a persisting myth, it's not because your diet contains too much cholesterol. The problem is in your liver where food is converted into the body's essential substances, including the right amount of so-called 'bad' LDL cholesterol. The series of chemical reactions is termed a metabolic pathway (like a production line). The speed at which this happens is controlled by an enzyme (a protein which speeds up a reaction without being destroyed) known as HMG CoA reductase (even that mouthful is an abbreviation). It controls the speed according to the amount of LDL cholesterol and other end products being formed. When there is sufficient LDL cholesterol the enzyme activity decreases. And vice versa.

It's just one example of a ubiquitous process in the body

known as negative feedback – not as in 'Unsatisfactory. Please repeat', more like 'That's enough for now, thanks. I'll let you know when I want more.'

Unfortunately, the enzyme can be kidded into 'thinking' it needs to speed things up thus producing too much LDL cholesterol causing arteries to fur up – hence the term 'bad' cholesterol. The enzyme is kidded by a diet too rich in the saturated fatty acids present in animal fats, especially dairy and fatty meat. Although you may know people who seem to be getting away with it, that does not disprove the concept: it simply means that their enzyme isn't so easily kidded or they have more circulating 'good' HDL-cholesterol stopping the arteries from furring up.

Not only animal fats but some vegetable fats like some of the palm oil found in many processed foods can put the bad LDL cholesterol up. Other culprits are the trans fats, liquid oils which have been solidified by hydrogenation to make them more acceptable to NW European tastes. As a rough guide, fats solid at room temperature are the ones to avoid while those liquid at room temperature are the best way of ensuring that you have enough fat in your diet.

So cream is okay because it is (to varying extents) a liquid then? No, because it owes its liquidity to its other non-fatty constituents. The same applies to full fat soft cheeses. For a clear and detailed account that dispels the myths surrounding the topic read the Harvard Medical School's Family Health Guide: The truth about fats: bad and good.[37]

Statins, developed from a fungal extract, have the opposite effect to saturated fats: they damp down the enzyme HMG CoA reductase. Not only are they the most powerful 'bad' LDL cholesterol reducers ever, more effective than diet alone, but they have direct beneficial effects on the arteries including those in the brain. But they, like other drugs, have side effects in some people and for borderline raised cholesterol their use should be preceded by a trial of diet change.[38]

*

We need an expert to tell us what specialists had been finding in their clinics at the time when Carl should have been referred, and how much benefit Carl might have obtained from timely correction of his vascular risk factors. After I've put all this stuff in the post for Ellie, I give her a ring.

PART 3

On Lawyers and Expert Witnesses

'Sir, I say that justice is truth in action.'

– Benjamin Disraeli, House of Commons, 1851

19

'I don't want this to happen to anyone else'
— Clinical negligence complainants

'Ellie, I don't know how you coped,' I say when she answers her phone.

'I didn't!' she says. 'I'm on anti-depressants. Me of all people!'

I know that loads of people would have gone under, even without their GP compounding the problem instead of solving it.

I explain that the doctors may not have been certain of the diagnosis, and even if they had felt sure they may well not have told them immediately in case they were wrong. But there's one thing I do know.

'What I *can* tell you is that they couldn't have ruled out dementia so they'd have kept him under specialist review,' I say.

Carl was only fifty-four then. They'd have ruled out treatable conditions like an under-active thyroid. Or a brain tumour needing urgent treatment. He would have had blood tests, psychological tests and a brain scan, probably an MRI scan, and been seen by a neurologist or a psychiatrist.

What, I wonder, would Carl and Ellie have done about the business with all this high-power clinical activity going on – and set to continue. I don't want to put words into her mouth by asking. I don't need to – she's read my thoughts.

'If that had happened, I'd have made sure Carl closed the business,' she tells me.

I wonder what astronomical figure the debts would have reached if Ellie hadn't taken action. And Ellie wonders again what they would have made of Carl at the Job Centre and when, if ever, Dr Bromwich would have cottoned on.

I explain how the management of early dementia has changed since we were students when the mainstay of treatment was nursing care like late stage dementia is now. As knowledge improved of how the brain works, a range of drugs became available that helped preserve brain function during the early stages before the disease takes hold. Drugs like the Galanthamine and Aricept which Carl benefited from. But they are merely helping with the brain's poor functioning that will cease eventually anyway.

It's a bit like taking tablets for a migraine: they can help if taken early enough in the attack but not if taken too late or for seriously disabling or very frequent attacks. You really need to find the underlying cause and deal with that.

Controlling the vascular risk is a more fundamental approach. I say that many top specialists had believed for some time that the progress of vascular dementia could be slowed in some cases but far too many NHS workers are still in the old mindset.

I tell Ellie it's rather technical, but I've sent her my thoughts on dementia and a book for carers[39] that should help make things clearer. She'll get the hang of it after she's read everything a time or two. I say I'm not the most appropriate authority to advise on whether dealing with Carl's vascular risk factors earlier might have helped slow down the progress of the dementia but I know people who are.

I ask her what Carl's consultant is like, knowing that she'd initiated the local research project on younger people with dementia 'to see if we can get something more for them'.

'She's lovely!' Ellie says, 'Nothing's too much trouble. All I've ever needed to do is leave a message with her secretary and she does her best for us. It's not her I'm complaining about.'

I'm sure Dr White would have been more than happy, had she seen Carl sooner, to have referred him to one of these experts even if it was only for Ellie to take comfort from knowing that everything possible was being done for Carl.

So where do we go from here, I wonder.

'What made you decide to complain?' I ask.

'Carl asked me to nail the bastards.'

I'd have done the same.

'I don't want this to happen to anyone else,' she says.

They all want that, I think.

'I wanted them to say sorry,' she says.

They all want that, I think.

'They wouldn't apologise,' I say, 'because they'd be scared of you coming on them for the £50,000.'

'So why did the Complaints Manager tell me to see my solicitor then? I'd get my day in court. Tell everybody the truth. And I'll give the £50,000 to the Alzheimer's Society,' she says.

They all want that, I think.

'It won't get to court. And you won't get £50,000.' I say.

I explain that you often get a phone call from the solicitor the afternoon beforehand saying they've reached a settlement for an amount that can feel like an insult. Both sides know you'll be forced to accept to stop it going to court, losing, then having to pay the defendant's costs.

'Should I go to the newspapers then?' she says.

'No, no, no!' I say, 'You can't do that. You'd be in big trouble.'

When she asks why, I say they could make it look as if she was taking out her anger over Carl's illness and the debts on the doctors who'd always done all they could to help. I tell her I'll see if I can find a clinical negligence solicitor who'll take a look at the case.

That's how we end up following another four-year trail leading into a farmyard full of barking dogs. And, through the upstairs window of the barn, there'll be a twelve-bore shotgun trained on us both.

20

No good shall come of this

I know of a firm of solicitors specialising in clinical negligence and personal injury. I hadn't had any dealings with them but I'd met the senior partner who'd helped me point someone I knew in the right direction – to good effect. I give him a ring.

The problem, I say, is that the GP continued beyond all professional reason to manage Carl's dementia as what he wrongly assumed was depression caused by business worries. If the GP had referred Carl to a specialist when he should, his business could have been closed when it was solvent instead of eight months later with debts which had escalated to £50,000.

He says there could be difficulties with that. He explains that the economic loss would have to result from the damage caused by the missed diagnosis for it to be actionable. Otherwise it's pure economic loss and not actionable. At least, I think that's what he's saying.

I explain that Carl's dementia had made him incapable of running the business that, for many years, had been a successful one. Carl should have been referred to a specialist between six months and a year after his first visit because, whatever the ultimate diagnosis, his worsening mental state was affecting his problem solving abilities when he had a big business decision to make with a deadline to meet, and it was affecting both their livelihoods and their marriage as his GP records show. This was about the time the debts began and over the ensuing months they escalated to £50,000. If the GP had taken the illness seriously instead of trivialising it they would have decided that the sensible thing to do was close Carl's business and live off the B&B.

Secondly, there are vascular risk factors like raised blood pressure, diabetes or raised cholesterol that need treating to avoid making any dementia worse. An appropriate expert would be needed to address the question of whether timely specialist management might have slowed the progress of his condition.

The senior partner rates the case provisionally as arguable as his written notes (which I won't find until years later) confirm. I send him the documentation plus my observations, including the name and contact details of a vascular diseases specialist. He's a doctor's doctor (knows his stuff) and a patient's doctor (makes you feel better). If he doesn't wish to give an opinion himself he'll certainly recommend someone else. I also enclose a copy of my C.V. including details of my qualifications (medical degree with a relevant specialist qualification in biochemical disorders e.g. diabetes and disorders of cholesterol metabolism), posts held, experience and research. Not outstanding but impressive enough.

The senior partner responds quickly, saying he's handing the case to the firm's head of clinical negligence. I have a vague sense of foreboding.

21

The shotgun is loaded

January 1999 – January 2000

About a month later, in the New Year of 1999, Ellie, Carl and I meet the head of clinical negligence, Caroline Archer. She is wearing a well-cut trouser suit, and is blonde, slim, and attractive with a gentle manner. Carl appreciates the purpose of the visit but doesn't join in the conversation. I too make no contribution. Most of the time is spent on finances.

Mrs Archer explains that she will apply for Legal Aid and obtain all Carl's GP and hospital records. Ellie says that there is no record in Carl's notes of her seeing the GP about Carl during the nine month gap in his visits. If there's nothing in her records either, the case might be dead in the water so we need to know now. Mrs Archer agrees and appears to make a note of it.

The interview ends with Mrs Archer saying that for the next few months she will be in overall charge from home with her assistant, Joan Baker, a nurse, doing the day-to-day handling. I feel uneasy, wondering how old her assistant is. Nursing training used to be practical and didactic but if she's a contemporary of Mrs Archer, it's more likely to be evidence based so there shouldn't be a problem.

At the beginning of July, Ellie phones me. She's just had a call from Joan Baker to say she's been granted Legal Aid and they're sending for the notes. She asks if I remember Mrs Archer agreeing that they needed her GP records as well as Carl's.

'She made a note of it, I'm sure. What's the problem?' I say.

Ellie tells me Joan Baker has explained, in a tone you'd use to a toddler, that it's Carl's notes which are required, not hers.

I wonder which of the two is running the case.

'How old did she sound on the phone?' I say.

'I'd guess in her mid-fifties,' Ellie says.

Old enough to be Mrs Archer's mother, I think. I feel more uneasy now.

Years later I will discover several things.

Mrs Archer's handwritten account of the meeting had included a note to obtain Ellie's GP records. But Joan Baker, whose job title is Medical Assistant, had logged her phone call to Ellie thus:

> *Client thinks she was told we would get her notes from GP*
> *as well.*
> *At some future date.*
> *File.*

Two attempts are made between July and Christmas 1999 to obtain Carl's hospital and GP records.

The solicitors' second demand for the hospital records is unnecessarily combative in tone: the solicitors had received and paid for them the previous month. They had even let Ellie know. And Ellie had always made it clear that she'd never had any quarrel whatsoever with Dr White's care – quite the reverse.

The first request for Carl's GP records was sent to the wrong GP (unconnected with the case, he is identifiable by his full name and address in another town) and they are paid for twice.

When Ellie receives her copy of Carl's GP records, I go through them. I find the reports of the blood tests taken at Carl's first visit. They were all normal apart from the cholesterol, the reason for its request being 'Routine test' i.e. unconnected with his current symptoms. The consultant chemical pathologist signing the form added the comment: 'Borderline TC [total cholesterol] and LDL [bad cholesterol]' underlining the values for emphasis.

This was evidence that Carl wasn't clearing his arteries, including those going to his brain, as well as he should. The result needed assessment in conjunction with Carl's other vascular risk factors.

Years later, I will realise, when trying to sort out chronology errors in the experts' reports (Chapters 27 and 30) which weaken the case, that the reason was Joan Baker's bizarre pagination error in Carl's GP records.

GP record cards, size A5, fit side-by-side in landscape orientation on a single sheet of A4 for photocopying. A reader seeing them thus arranged would expect to find page one of the GP notes on the left side of the first A4 page with page two on the right. Page three of the GP notes should be on the left side of the second A4 page and page four on the right. And so on.

Instead Joan Baker placed pages one and three of the GP notes side-by-side on the first A4 sheet, pages two and four of the GP notes side-by-side on the second sheet – and so on. Alternate, instead of consecutive, pages side-by-side on the same sheet *throughout Carl's GP records from 1972 onwards. It wasn't a one-off mistake.*

Ellie could make neither head nor tail of this novel sequence of Carl's visits to the doctor from 1962 onwards. She cut the A4 pages in half in order to return the GP notes to their original order. Reluctant to do anything so drastic to a legal document, I achieved the same result less conveniently by numbering each GP page according to the visit dates in the margin.

I believe this was when the twelve-bore shotgun was first loaded.

22

Who's running the show?

January 2000 – July 2000

Our meeting with Mrs Archer in mid-January 2000 gets off to a shaky start. She says the gap with no visits between Carl's first visit in August 1990 and his next visit in September 1991 weakens the case.

Ellie points out Carl's two follow-up visits in autumn 1990 in Carl's GP records when the GP failed to monitor the cognitive defects. Remembering Joan Baker's dismissive comment to Ellie about her own notes, I say I thought we'd agreed a year ago that we needed them to confirm her crucial visit to the GP in March 1991. That would make two, possibly three, documented visits during the gap.

Mrs Archer asks Ellie to sign an application for her GP records before she leaves.

Mrs Archer tells me she finds my initial observations for the senior partner very helpful. I am used to such comments. The outcome in my previous cases has always been according to my report, irrespective of whether it supported the view of the party who had engaged me. I'm ready for the inevitable cross questioning – but it doesn't happen. She doesn't even ask me to suggest questions for the experts in what is a complex case.

Oh well, I think, it's up to her, she knows what she's doing. But I'm feeling very uneasy now.

Ellie tells Mrs Archer about the local research project showing that only Carl and two others were diagnosed late prompting her complaint to the health authority. If Carl had been undergoing specialist tests by the same time as most of the others were, they'd have known something was wrong and sold the business before the debts escalated. Ellie says she will send Mrs Archer a copy.

Mrs Archer asks about Carl's business finances. Ellie explains that his accountant is now aged seventy-six and in poor health. His clients' files, including Carl's, were taken over by another firm when he retired and would normally be kept for ten years after Carl's business closed in March 1992. Ellie agrees to send contact details for both the accountant and a member of Carl's staff who had been worried about the change in him, and all the bank statements she has for the business. They are complete from January 1990, eight months before Carl's first visit to the GP to four years later when the debts were paid off and the account closed.

Years later, I uncover this sequence of events (my italics):

19th January 2000 Ellie sends accountant's and employee's contact details.

9th February 2000 Joan Baker's file note: 'Mrs Archer *now* wants Mrs Valente's GP records.'

15th February 2000 Joan Baker's note on Ellie's phone call asking about her GP records: 'Client told they haven't arrived because the request has only recently been made. *Request hasn't gone out yet because letter isn't on the new system.*'

16th February 2000 Mrs Archer requests Ellie's records.

18th February 2000 Ellie sends Carl's bank statements plus details of having to use her one-third share from the sale of her deceased mother's house, her childhood home, to pay off some of the debts. She's added a footnote in red felt tip: 'MAM'S HOUSE. MY MONEY. £10,000. GONE.'

25th February 2000 Mrs Archer's file note: 'Client sent me a lot of financial figures. I think that these are Carl's but they do not seem to make much sense in isolation. I will have to look through them in more detail when I have time.'

7th March 2000 Joan Baker's file note: 'Awaiting Mrs Valente's GP records.'

8th March 2000 Joan Baker's file note: '*Mrs Valente's GP records arrive*; paginated, sorted, read.'

19th April 2000 Mrs Archer writes to Ellie: (a) acknowledges receipt of 'detailed information' sent on 18th February (b) explains that she will be amending Ellie's statement *once she has received her GP records*.

July 2000 The accountant dies.

There is no record of the solicitors ever contacting the accountant, obtaining Carl's business accounts or looking again at the bank statements.

I add a postscript in red felt tip: 'CARL'S WISH. ELLIE'S PROMISE. EVIDENCE. GONE.'

23

'Shoot the messenger'

Summer 2000

Ellie phones me. She is very upset. After she's told me about it so am I. And full of guilt. One evening while they were on holiday in Spain two weeks earlier, Carl had become confused and aggressive. After emergency treatment, he was flown home by air ambulance and admitted to hospital. Acute urinary retention had caused a toxic confusional state.

Poor Carl, I think. As if his dementia isn't enough. But I don't think poor Ellie. 'Why did you take him abroad?' I ask. Pause. I could have bitten my tongue off.

'Because,' she says, 'Carl's always loved holidays in the sun. He was really enjoying it until then. I told the people at our table right away about Carl's dementia and they were all really kind.'

'I'm sorry,' I say.

'It's okay,' she says. And tells me I'm the only person – apart from Carl's consultant who's lovely – who understands. Others ignore or blame her for what's happened: the carer's double whammie. But I still don't deserve her response.

'Is it his prostate?' I ask.

She says it's a recurrence of a problem cured until now by an operation in 1976. The surgeon, who'd said at the time he would see Carl again whenever he needed, saw him and told Ellie how sad he was to see this man who'd been one of his most rewarding cases reduced to a shadow of his former self. He also queried whether Carl's dementia

104

could be caused by new variant Creutzfeldt-Jakob disease (mad cow disease) because he used to be a butcher. I sense he was clutching at diagnostic straws as a way of comforting Ellie with his concern.

Then the day care staff told her that Carl was crawling about on his hands and knees all day and they couldn't stop him. He'd have to go into full-time care if he couldn't be stopped. She took Carl home hoping familiar surroundings would help but they didn't. Round and round on his hands and knees all day and she couldn't stop him either. He's now in full-time nursing care together with his pension and benefits. She is left alone to support herself in a six-bedroom house.

'Can we tell if Carl's got CJD?' she asks.

I find it hard to be explicit. 'Well, uh, no,' I say, 'it's either a brain biopsy or, uh, a post-mortem, depending...' Nobody would do a brain biopsy on a patient in Carl's condition. And if Carl died it would need a specialist's post-mortem to test for CJD. I write to Mrs Archer, sending a copy to Ellie, to explain but by the time the letter arrives, Ellie has already phoned them.

Years later I will read Joan Baker's log of that phone call:

22 May 2000. Between illness + job + CJD [sic] *If he died would PM be forced and biased to prevent full diagnosis. Her cousin says he needs a brain biopsy.*

I imagine, too late to set the record straight, the comments that would have whipped around the solicitors' tea-room – and how much further afield I'll never know:

Brain biopsy on a poor chap in that state? She's the one who needs her head examined! She's ignorant. She should be struck off! With friends like that the client doesn't need enemies!

Good job I'd retired by then, I think – because the twelve-bore shotgun had been fired at me.

24

'I swear by Almighty God ...'

Spring 2000

Years later I find four different statements of what Ellie will swear to in court. Only one, probably the second, with Ellie's amendments in the margins, is signed and dated (11th February 2000). Five days later Mrs Archer writes to Ellie:

> *I have prepared a more detailed statement on your behalf...*
> *When I receive your GP notes we may have to make further*
> *amendments to your statement.*

After these amendments, described later by Mrs Archer as 'quite heavy', the statement will go to Ellie for checking and signing. *There is no record of that happening. Two of the experts note that the copy they received is unsigned and undated.* They must have received either a later one that was never sent to Ellie for signing or one the solicitor had made earlier.

Ellie seems to have corrected only those errors and omissions which she understood. There is a confusing paragraph about Carl's response to the anti-dementia drug Galanthamine – two years after he was being cared for by a specialist about whom Ellie had no complaints at all.

This sentence on Galanthamine characterises the statement:

> *...I am aware from the medical records however that*
> *the perceptual improvements* are not supported *by the*

formalized [correct word is formal] *test results which showed very poor overall memory functioning...*

I've known Ellie since we were kids. It's not how she speaks or writes. I can't imagine her using an adjective like perceptual. Carl's hospital records have both him and Ellie saying he is more cheerful on the Galanthamine and doing jobs around the house better. The improvements *were supported* by two consultant psychiatrists and the observations of the consultant psychologist who did the tests. This misleading sentence exemplifies Mrs Archer's concern over the standard of Carl's hospital care which is not the basis of the complaint.

The paragraph on Carl's business failure reads:

> *During this time the business started to fail as my husband clearly was not capable of continuing to manage the business. I believe it finally collapsed in March/April 1992.*

I would not have expected Ellie to use a word like 'clearly' at a time when she was bewildered by their GP's trivialisation of Carl's illness. But she could have expected a hard time in court on the use of the words 'clearly' and 'believe':

> *Let me turn, Mrs Valente, if I may, to 1991 when it became clear to you that your husband was incapable of running the business, and yet you did nothing, even being unsure of the date when your unfortunate husband's business collapsed...Oh, I see, it only became clear to you later... May I remind you, Mrs Valente, that this is a court of law and you are on oath...*

Equally unfortunate is this sentence:

Had an earlier diagnosis been made, my husband and I would have been granted the opportunity to receive the appropriate medication for his condition and to therefore prevent such serious degeneration.

It is an unwarranted exaggeration of my measured explanation to both Ellie and the solicitors of current thinking on vascular dementia.

There are other significant errors and omissions:

1. There is no mention of the 1991 regulations which forced Carl to reorganise his business.
2. Ellie's break from running her successful B&B at a difficult time in Carl's illness is labelled her business failure. It wasn't. It was successful enough to pay off Carl's massive business debts and she closed it in a planned and rational manner about five years after Carl died.
3. Ellie's note in the margin of the signed statement about their son's advice to close the business when he saw 'the state *the business* was in' was *inaccurately transcribed thus:* 'The business was closed as soon as he realised the extent of *his father's deterioration.*'
4. Ellie's note about Carl's business debt, *her main contention,* in the margin of the only signed statement is omitted.

Her statement of what she will swear to in court is not what she said to anyone who would listen.

25

'I'm in charge!'
– Bruce Forsyth

May – October 2000

In May Mrs Archer tells Ellie that she has asked for a report from a GP, Dr Cooper, and they should hear from her soon. Our meeting with Mrs Archer to discuss the report takes place in October, after Ellie's four failed attempts during August to find out what is happening.

Years after the case ends I discover the sequence of events leading up to the meeting.

Mrs Archer sends the first instruction letter to Dr Cooper on May 19th. She phones Dr Cooper on 6 September, presumably as a result of Ellie's queries, to ask her to expedite the report. The next day she prepares another letter of instruction to Dr Cooper which she sends two weeks later with the same enclosures as the 19th May letter plus an extra item.

It is my commentary for the senior partner on the correct GP management of cognitive impairment showing how the GP's conduct had fallen below the standard you would reasonably expect. The letter crosses in the post with Dr Cooper's report. Dr Cooper writes to Mrs Archer:

> *You will by now be aware that I have already prepared a report...I proceeded after our telephone conversation when you asked me to expedite the report. I acted according to your instructions of 20 May 2000. The materials appear*

to be duplicates apart from the additional commentary. The questions you ask me are to some extent different although covering the same issues. Please let me know what you wish me to do.

Mrs Archer replies on 11 October:

...I am sorry if I confused you by sending out duplicate instructions – a draft set must have been retained on file and sent out in error...

But the duplicate instructions weren't a retained draft set from May: they were prepared in September, *the day after Mrs Archer's request to expedite the report as her own notes show.*

A week later Mrs Archer replies again: '...Unfortunately there was a mix-up at this end. Please ignore the second letter.'

There are pages missing from the single copy of the instruction letter in the solicitor's documents: (1) its last page has 'contd' in the bottom right hand corner (2) *there are no questions for the expert in it* (3) there are neat staple holes at the same place in all the pages which have then been re-stapled together.

What was all that about, I'll always wonder.

When Ellie and I meet Mrs Archer, she is surprised to find Ellie hasn't been sent a copy and asks Joan Baker to print two copies.

It's the first time we've met Mrs Baker. She is grey-haired, in her fifties, and her dress is not quite smart casual. She hands a copy to Ellie, slaps the other down in front of me and, with a toss of her head, leaves the room.

I skim read the report whilst listening to Mrs Archer going through it with Ellie. Dr Cooper's conclusions are the same as mine: the GP's management of the case was unacceptable. She draws particular attention to the GP's consistent failure to check on cognitive function; his failure to act on the evidence from both patient and his close associate of business and marital difficulties caused by the cognitive decline; the importance of identifying its serious/treatable causes in a middle-aged man; determining the patient's functioning level to help them plan their lives. I'm over the moon when I read this. The expert sees it like we do.

I focus on the page Mrs Archer and Ellie have reached.

'There's a problem with the dates,' I say.

Mrs Archer looks across at me. She's frowning, her neat lips pursed.

'Dr Payne,' she says, 'I read this report carefully before you arrived.'

I wasn't in that fortunate position, of course, so I check the dates now. Thanks to Joan Baker's pagination error, Dr Cooper has listed Carl's visits in the autumn of 1992 and 1993 together as if they'd all occurred in autumn 1992. Still, according to Mrs Archer, there is no mistake.

I know there must be. According to his medical records, Carl went on Hydergine, an anti-dementia drug, on his consultant's recommendation, in autumn *1993*. According to the mistake, Carl was put on it in autumn *1992* by the GP for the dementia he didn't know Carl had.

So, I wonder, couldn't the defence try muddying the waters by claiming that the delay in starting Carl's treatment was a year less than it really was, therefore insufficient to be negligent. Mrs Archer, barely convinced, agrees to ask Dr Cooper to reconsider the relevant paragraphs of the report. I sense she is taken aback by Dr Cooper's conclusion that the management of Carl's case was unacceptable.

We move on to the final topic: choosing an appropriate expert to advise on the effects of the missed diagnosis.

'For pre-senile dementia,' I say, 'a neurologist…'

Raising her hand, palm facing towards me, fingertips pointing upwards, Mrs Archer cuts me short: 'I am perfectly capable of instructing my own experts.'

26

Chinese whispers

After leaving the solicitor, Ellie asks me in an uncertain tone what I think.

You couldn't rate the meeting as friendly but, hyped up by Dr Cooper's opinion, I'm in no mood to worry.

'So far, so good,' I say, 'we're on to the next stage.'

Ellie says nothing.

Years later I read Mrs Archer's handwritten notes during the meeting, and her typed version dated for later that day.

Mrs Archer's handwritten notes:

> *Cholesterol – done at same time Sep 90.* [Carl's first visit]
> *'Borderline total cholesterol and* ['bad'] *LDL cholesterol – consultant chemical pathologist's annotation.* [He's also underlined the values for emphasis]
> *Essentially normal' – Dr Cooper's report*

Dr Cooper was referring to the blood tests to check for the effect of Carl's heavy drinking at that time. The cholesterol done at the same time was a routine check: it says so in the REASON FOR REQUEST box on the form. The consultant chemical pathologist, an expert in these matters, is commenting on the cholesterol test done in his own laboratory. His initialled annotation was to draw the GP's attention to a cholesterol result that required evaluation and *not* be written off as normal. I should know: I've added enough such comments myself in my time as a specialist. The rationale is clearly explained in Bhatnagar and Durrington's 1989 review article.[40]

Mrs Archer's typed notes (later that day):

> *We discussed the cholesterol levels – it was taken during 1990 and an annotation is made on that by the consultant chemical pathologist to confirm that the levels were essentially normal.*

What? I don't remember, nor would I have taken part in, any such discussion. More important, for the sake of truth, Mrs Archer's own handwritten notes during the meeting a few hours earlier show that the chemical pathologist's annotation highlights the fact that the cholesterol levels were *not* essentially normal.

Before I retired I would have used the interesting comparison of Carl's results with Ellie's as a teaching point. Her total cholesterol is significantly higher than Carl's. So she's more likely than Carl to have a heart attack or a stroke, right?

Wrong. Ellie has a well above average amount of 'good' cholesterol in her circulation keeping her arteries clear and that raises her total cholesterol level. But her 'bad' LDL cholesterol is higher than ideal too. It's the balance between good and bad cholesterol that matters. And there are other vascular risk factors to take into account in the individual patient: Body Mass Index, blood pressure, gender, smoking and personal and family history.

There are computer formulae now that give due weight to all these risk factors in predicting vascular disorders like heart attacks and strokes, the one recommended by NICE being available at qrisk.org.[41] They would have shown that Ellie's risk at the time, despite her higher total cholesterol than Carl's, was around half the female average whilst Carl's risk was almost double the male average. And – this point is worth labouring – even in 1991 before the days of computer formulae there were UK specialists in vascular disorders (including vascular dementia) highly skilled in the art of applying their science to cases like Carl's.

Mrs Archer's typed note continues:

> *The cholesterol levels were being done to consider the differential diagnosis...*

No! They weren't because:

1. They were a routine test: *it says so on the request form* (see above).
2. The GP didn't have a differential diagnosis: he had one wrong diagnosis – depression. *That's the crux of the case.*

The next paragraph is on another discussion that I don't remember: the choice of specialist expert. I only recall Mrs Archer's peremptory gesture when I'd tried to point out that a neurologist with an interest in dementia would be the expert of choice for a case of early-onset dementia.

Mrs Archer's opinion is that the choice of expert should be on a like-for-like basis – in Carl's case a psychiatrist with a particular interest in dementia. However, the next sentence negates her own logic: 'We have to use a standard jobbing psychiatrist. Mrs Valente agreed with this analysis and gave instructions that I should instruct an appropriate expert.'

The expert of Mrs Archer's choice will prove to be none of these.

27

Under new management

October 2000 – September 2001

Years later I will piece together from solicitors' records what went on behind the scenes during the eleven months' wait for the psychiatrist's report.

Despite several telephone calls, Ellie hears nothing from the solicitors until in March 2001 her phone call is taken by another solicitor, Mrs Carter. She has been brought in to clear the backlog of work. The psychiatrist has not yet confirmed his willingness to provide a report.

Having heard nothing, Ellie complains on 18th April about the lack of progress, with written confirmation to the senior partner. Her call provokes frenetic action that day by Mrs Carter. She:

1. Phones the psychiatrist who says he would expect to complete a report by mid/end-June.
2. Sends him a letter of instruction with eight questions (which seem to have wandered from Ellie's original complaint), warning him to take care to avoid being misled by the confusing dates in Carl's GP records.
3. Emails Mrs Archer at her home with copy to the senior partner.
4. Writes to Dr Cooper about confusion on dates in her report (Chapter 27) asking her to amend her report as necessary.
5. Updates Ellie.

A week later the psychiatrist, Dr Forrester, phones Mrs Carter to say that it was clearly a late diagnosis. A month later Dr Cooper sends an amended report that doesn't affect her overall conclusions. She shows how Joan Baker's pagination error in Carl's GP notes had caused the confusion.

In mid-June, having heard nothing, Ellie tells Mrs Carter that she is considering moving to another firm. I manage to dissuade her because it's generally not a good idea to change solicitors and we are so close to an answer now it makes sense to hang on. Mrs Carter hears from Dr Forrester that he will be unable to complete the report before the end of July due to pressure of work, updates Ellie, explains that she will be leaving soon, and wishes Ellie 'all the very best of luck' with her claim.

Dr Forrester's report arrives in mid-August. Mrs Archer makes some notes:

> *This is just a preliminary reading just to give me a feel for it...we are going to be very hard pushed to succeed in a claim here as there is no evidence that earlier diagnosis could have arrested the development of this condition.* [What about the business and marital problems and the effect of the debts?] *Also there is really no time window when the GP should have made an earlier diagnosis/ referral.* [The six month time window is 25th March 1991 – 25th September 1991]

A week later (September 18th) Mrs Archer writes to Dr Forrester:

> *Thank you so much for sending through your report. I am sorry that I was not able to get back to you via the telephone but I have hardly been in the office recently...*

28

Alice in expertland

September 18th 2001
Ellie rings.

'He says I'm a basket case.' If she wasn't shouting, I know she'd be crying.

I wonder if it's the neighbour who's apt to park across her drive.

'No, not him! I can cope with him.'

I'm worried that she's getting near the edge. The carer's become another patient. And now that Carl's in full-time care and he's begun suffering from fits as well, she's hanging on to him by an unravelling thread.

Who could be saying she's a basket case? A nasty suspicion comes into my mind. Surely not, I think. Dr Cooper's report was in our favour.

'I've got this letter from the solicitor...we haven't got a case... the psychiatrist says Dr Bromwich didn't diagnose the dementia in time because we're both basket cases...it's an insult. We're not basket cases,' she says.

'Course you're not,' I say.

'He's not an expert. He's ignorant. He doesn't know what TATT means. Even I know it means tired all the time,' she says.

What? I think. A doctor who doesn't know what TATT means? I worry that the report will not 'enable the trier of facts to understand the facts in question'.[42]

She sends me a copy. I read the covering letter first:

> ...*it would be best if you could read through the report carefully and then make an appointment to meet with me to discuss it...it would seem that we will not be able to succeed with a claim. I am basing this assertion on the psychiatrist's views that even with an earlier diagnosis, the cause of the deterioration could not have been prevented or arrested.*

So a claim for pecuniary loss caused by failure to evaluate a complaint of severe cognitive decline won't succeed because its cause could not have been prevented or arrested.

I can't get my head round this so I turn to Dr Forrester's report. His C.V. consists of this sentence: Consultant Psychiatrist approved under section 12(2) of the Mental Health Act 1983.

Uh-oh! He's taken the case on without declaring a particular interest in dementia. So, compared with Carl's psychiatrist, the local dementia specialist, he's an *un*like-for-like psychiatrist.

He has failed to heed Mrs Carter's warning about the confusing dates in Carl's GP records. He writes:

> *The only consistent finding is urinary tract problems from 1976 onwards.*

What? I think. I check Carl's GP records. The urinary tract problems (severe chronic retention causing recurrent urinary infections) began in spring *1974* and were *cured* in July 1976 for another twenty-odd years by bladder neck surgery. The problems didn't *begin* in 1976, they *ended*.

Probably a typo, I think, and continue reading.

I come to the heading 'Psychiatric History until 1990'. What psychiatric history, I wonder? The one that his wife, family, friends, colleagues, Carl's four GPs and his two specialists, and Dr Cooper (the GP expert) didn't believe he had. The purported psychiatric history consists of six episodes from 1972 onwards. I quickly discount four.

In 1972 and 1979 Carl had two brief self-limiting periods of fatigue and stress such as might occur in anyone, especially a workaholic businessman.

In 1981, there was a GP investigation of possible cardio-vascular disease needing two follow-up visits in which a slightly raised blood pressure was recorded. Carl, then aged forty-four with two very bright teenage sons to see through university, had good reason to be concerned about cardiovascular disease: his own father had died aged fifty-six of a heart attack when Carl was twenty-one.

In 1987 he had a self-limiting skin problem which could, in him, have been occupational.

Dr Forrester's transcript of the remaining episodes under the psychiatric history heading reads:

> _April 1975_. _General malaise._ [TATT: which I understand
>   to indicate an exaggerated presentation? totally above
>   the top?] _Irritable and tense. Surmontil 25 mgm_
>   _x 2 nocte._ [anti-depressant]
> _May 1979_ _Overtired. No physical symptoms. Reassured._
> _9th June 1975_. _OK mentally now._

The May visit actually occurred in _1979 as stated._ It is not an inconsequential scrivener's error. It appears where it does _thanks to Mrs Baker's pagination error._ But together with the omission of the slightly raised blood pressure on that visit, the reader's impression could be of _three_ consultations in three months in _1975_ for vague psychiatric symptoms with no physical abnormalities.

Likewise, his incomplete transcripts of the April and June 1975 visits appear to be for vague symptoms for which an anti-depressant was prescribed. The full transcript of the GP's notes of the urinary tract problems from their start in spring 1974 to their cure in July 1976, including the April and June 1975 entries, reads (omitted items are in italics):

- *6.9.74 intermittent febrile episodes* [high temperature] *before and after cholera jab. Frequency* [of urination] *Nocturia x 2* [getting up in night twice]. *O/E Slight tender L loin* [possible urinary infection extending to left kidney] *Urine sample to lab. Start antibiotic.*
- *17.9.74 Loins no pain or tenderness. Lab confirms urinary infection: antibiotic changed NB Sister died of TB kidney in 1951.*
- 29.4.75 General malaise/TATT/irritable and tense. *No urinary symptoms this time BP 130/80. Loins not tender. Urine specimen to lab.* [GP rightly querying urine infection] Surmontil 25mg x 2 nocte [anti-depressant].
- 9.6.75 *OK until 2 days ago – back pain, febrile* [has temperature]. OK mentally now. *Urine to lab.* [GP rightly querying urine infection]
- 14.4.76 *Dysuria again* [pain on urination] *Frequency/ nocturia Backache* [signs of urinary infection possibly extending to kidneys] *Urine to lab, septrin* [antibiotic for urinary infection] *refer to surgeon*
- July 1976 *Bladder neck resection*

Unfortunately, the above oversights plus the 1976 cure date being mistaken for the 1974 start date of the urinary tract problems, lend themselves to the conclusion that these were psychiatric episodes.

Carl must have been feeling pretty under the weather for these two years: tests showed that his chronic urine retention amounted to between half and one litre. Half to one kilogram is a heavy weight, whether sterile or infected, to be carting around in your lower abdomen all day.

His twenty-seven-year-old sister's death from TB of the kidney could have been a weight on his mind as well. Carl was thirty-seven at the time with a wife and two young sons to support. That may have been the GP's thinking behind the prescription of the two month course of an anti-depressant.

The common medical acronym TATT means 'tired all the time'. I am unaware of any other meanings. Chronic severe urinary retention with recurrent urinary infections cured in 1976 by major surgery isn't part of a psychiatric history.

I recognised, from the notes and the tone of the doctors' correspondence, that the relief of Carl's urinary tract problem was one of those rewarding outcomes that you'll always look back on. But now it's overshadowed for the surgeon by his sorrow on seeing how dementia had all but destroyed his former patient.

29

Muddied waters

In the next section, 'Wife's concerns during this period', he notes 'that she herself has a history of anxiety dating back to July 1962 when she was treated with Stelazine 1 mgm twice daily.'

Uh-oh! We're back in 1962 via a history of anxiety that nobody in the family has ever heard of. I've known Ellie since we were in the infants' school. It doesn't fit. She's always been up-front with all her feelings. No psychological problems after the babies were born, a rough guide to psychological stability.

A month's supply of Stelazine was prescribed with no follow-up visit and no reason given for the consultation. It could have been for either stress or a stomach upset. It is not part of a psychiatric history.

The next item is this:

In April 1980 she was described as TATT, irritable and tense.

Who in eighteen years doesn't feel tired, irritable, and tense at times? It was when Carl's business was flourishing, they owned a block of flats with tenants, and the boys were teenagers still at home. The GP, knowing the patient, didn't rate it. It's not a psychiatric diagnosis.

Next comes this:

On 25th March 1981 it is evident that she was 'concerned about husband's mental health, had a spell of anxiety

*and depression about 6 months ago, she says he is making
mistakes and poor concentration'.*

Ellie didn't see the doctor at all in March 1981 although she saw him
three times that year about the usual things. The full transcript reads:

> *Concerned about husband's mental health. Had spell
> of anxiety/depression about 6 months ago. She says he's
> making mistakes + poor concentration. Leading to friction:
> business marital. Getting anxious + sleep less good –
> diff. getting off. Did stop HRT because weight gain – but
> sweats resumed & therefore started again. Discussion.
> See husband.*

The psychiatrist has got the date wrong, giving it as 25th March
1981, not 25th March *1991*.

So it's a typo, a scrivener's error. But it isn't inconsequential.
It appears from the wrong date that Ellie's complaints about her
husband's behaviour *preceded his first symptoms of dementia by nine
years.* Together with the psychiatrist's omission of the GP's note on
business and marital friction, and of the GP's declared intention to
'See husband', the reader might assume that the GP had assessed
Ellie as a moaning menopausal wife complaining about little more
than her husband leaving his dirty socks on the bedroom carpet.

Next comes this paragraph:

> *Her statement indicates that she had expressed her concern
> about her husband's mental faculties, especially his
> inability to continue with the business to her GP on several
> occasions, notably March 1991, summer 1991, February
> 1992 and March 1992. This concern was written in the
> GP notes in specific and clear terms only in November
> 1992, although he noted Mrs Valente's concern about her
> husband's general state of mental health in March 1991.*

Dr Forrester is mistaken. As we have seen, Ellie's concern was recorded by the GP in specific and clear enough terms (business and marital problems) for him to make a note to 'See husband' at the consultation *on 25th March 1991* – the one he transcribed as *March 1981*.

He continues:

> *Her stress was both subjective and objective, and in view of her history* [what history?], *the GP has reasonably, in my view, given her anti-depressants and referred her to the counselling service.*

We're heading into the next farmyard full of barking dogs.

30

'What I tell you three times is true'
– Lewis Carroll, 1832–1898

Still under 'Wife's concerns during this period' there's this:

> *The GP's management of him to that point* [what point?]
> *is also reasonable in view of his history of affective problems*
> *in the past, his response to the anti-depressant medication.*

The GP's management was *un*reasonable: irrespective of whether Carl's increasing cognitive decline had been accompanied or preceded by his or his wife's psychiatric problems, it called for urgent specialist investigation. And a patient with a depressive history is as 'entitled' to develop dementia as anyone else, possibly more so according to some studies.

Dr Forrester makes the important point elsewhere in his report that the improvement in Carl's mood (with anti-depressants) was not accompanied by a retrieval of his concentration ability (indicative of dementia rather than depression). Unfortunately, he does not develop this argument further, simply referring again to what he describes as Carl's history of 'affective' problems. But he has said it twice now.

Under 'Discussion':

> *Pre-senile dementia can encompass a variety of aetiolo-*
> *gies, most commonly multiple infarcts, Arteriosclerotic or*
> *Alzheimer. It is virtually impossible to arrive at a definitive*

diagnosis as to which precise pathology is causing the demen-
tia since the clinical picture of all three common courses tend
to overlap and clinical terms they share and present with
progressive cognitive deterioration. [sic]

It goes without saying that making a definitive, as opposed to the
normal presumptive, diagnosis of the dementia type is virtually
impossible without a post-mortem or brain biopsy.

He continues:

There was a history of episodic presentation with anxiety
and depression in 1972, 1975, 1979, 1981 and 1987
before he presented to his GP in August 1990 with poor
concentration and memory. It is not unreasonable then
for the GP to perceive his illness as one of an affective
[psychiatric] *nature…his wife had expressed her concern*
about her husband's mental abilities, but that was
attributed [by whom?] at least to some extent if not
predominantly to her own anxiety and depression…

He has said it three times.

He continues:

…pre-senile dementia, particularly of the Alzheimer's
type tends to follow a progressive course, and no specific
treatment including Hydergine or Donepezil have
proved to be capable of reversing or slowing down such
progress regardless of the stage at which the patient is
referred to the specialist service the advantage of early
referral of course is the initiation of the support services
e.g. day centre OT, and the start of investigations
to eliminate reversible aetiological causes, e.g. space
occupying lesion. [sic]

He has cited none of the literature in mainstream and specialist peer-reviewed journals nor given the reasons for his opinion.

And, on page 14, this:

> *It is conceivable that a referral in 1991 may have resulted in the identification of a very early dementing process and then it would have been theoretically possible for Mr Valente and his family to negotiate the business problem at an earlier stage. I must say however that a definitive diagnosis would have been very difficult to arrive at that stage.*

It goes without saying that a definitive diagnosis would have been impossible then. The point about diagnosis is that dementia *could not have been excluded* so Carl should have been kept under specialist review starting between 26th March 1991 and 25th September 1991 thus enabling them to negotiate the business problem in the light of that and prevent the massive debts. It's as simple as that.

Dr Forrester has not answered the pivotal question that was his, as the specialist expert, to answer: whether, on the balance of probability, the cognitive defects (trivialised by the GP) were, by their nature (impaired numeracy, concentration and memory) and/or severity, the explanation for the mess Carl got the business into.

In his role as the specialist expert witness, he has zeroed-in on various psychological aspects of the case, but with errors and omissions, and without evaluating the contrary views of Ellie's and Carl's own doctors.

We have arrived in the farmyard full of barking dogs, with a twelve-bore shotgun trained on us from the barn window, and the case stuck in limbo.

31

The sound of gunfire

Years later, I find Dr Forrester's covering letter to Mrs Archer enclosing his report. He apologises for the delay, regrets not having had 'a little discussion with you on the telephone' beforehand, and says that he phoned Ellie the day before finishing his report. The rest makes disturbing reading:

> *In addition to my report, I am enclosing a summary of his medical history, encompassing extracts from his wife's medical history for your own reference.*

In his role as the specialist expert witness, he has zeroed-in on various psychological aspects of the case, but with errors and omissions, and without evaluating the contrary views of Ellie's and Carl's own doctors.

There's no sign of the summary now. Why wasn't it included in his report? And how does a summary of someone's medical history 'encompass' extracts from the spouse's medical history? What does he mean? He continues:

> *You will see that their medical histories are quite intertwined* [how?] *and should this case proceed to court, I can well imagine the cross examination process and the defence relating the GP's responses to his wife's requests and concerns not only to her husband but to her own state of*

health bearing in mind her own history ie personal and family. This is important as her statement may lead to an impression that the GP was misconstruing her concerns, and that would be correct since she had her own difficulties as well as her observations and legitimate concerns about her husband. I did not intend this summary of the records to be disclosed and do not consider it a part of my report. It is intended for your information only as a backdrop to my own conclusions.'

If relevant to the case, a professional assessment of it belonged in his report. If not, it belonged nowhere. If he was in doubt, say, about something that might come out in court, it was up to the solicitor to raise the matter with the client. But there is no record of any phone calls or emails from Dr Forrester to Mrs Archer so we'll never know whether she ever discovered what was being hinted at in a covering letter which the client and his Litigation Friend were unaware of.

Shots had been fired at Ellie and the case was almost lost.

32

We have our say

November 2001

I have put together a commentary. Due to lack of time it's not pruned and polished to the standard of an expert report but it's coherent enough for a trained legal mind.

It comprises:

1. Comments on Dr Forrester's report.
2. Challenge of Mrs Archer's assertion that a claim cannot succeed on the basis of Dr Forrester's view that even with an earlier diagnosis the cause of the deterioration could not have been prevented or arrested.
3. Criticisms of Mrs Baker's document preparation notably the pagination error.
4. Evidence of the interest my research on lipid abnormalities (vascular risk factors as we have seen) had attracted outside my own profession and country.
5. My observations on how the case should have been handled.
6. A note on the case of possible dementia that turned out, thanks to my timely investigation, to be treatable thyroid disease so he was able to return to his job (see Chapter 12).

Ellie forwards it immediately to Mrs Archer with a covering letter:

Ref. your letter of 18 Sept 01 and copy of psychiatrist's report.

I fail to understand why you chose to use the services of a man who obviously has a problem with the English language! TATT means "tired all the time" not totally above the top. I am most indignant at his perception of my mental state. I was a Samaritan volunteer for 3 yrs. I was on the executive committee of our local Tourism Association and recently been voted on to the executive committee of our local carers' association. I have run two businesses whilst caring for a sick husband. Does this sound like a woman with a mental history? Could I please see the list supplied by the Legal Aid Board from which you chose the 'so-called expert'. The Legal Aid Board should be made aware of his difficulty with the English language.

Please find enclosed a report done by my cousin which I feel is nearer the truth than anything your man has come up with.

Please read it and I await your comments.

January 2002 Mrs Archer replies:

I am quite aware that Dr Forrester has misunderstood the medical abbreviation TATT and I have obviously pointed this out to him and asked if this changes his opinion. I have also exchanged the reports between Dr Cooper and Dr Forrester and asked for their comments on the issues arising insofar as they are relevant to their own discipline.

Dr Forrester is an expert who was recommended by the organisation who run the most authoritative countrywide database of experts specialising in clinical negligence. I have no hesitation in recommending their screening of experts to you but at the same time, this is only effective when feedback is given and I have completed the appropriate

131

> *feedback sheet commenting on his misconstruction of this basic medical term.*
>
> *I have to say that it is inaccurate for you to suggest that the psychiatrist is anything other than an independent expert whose first duty is to the court, not to you or indeed to me and he has to prepare the report with this obligation in mind.*
>
> *I think it would be most appropriate to await the comments of our two experts and then for us to meet. I anticipate a conference may elucidate many of these issues.*
>
> *Before Conference, it is appropriate for us to deal with the financial implications of this case so that our barrister can advise accordingly. To this end, I would be grateful if you would please let me have details of the business insofar as you are able. I will need the completed business accounts and insofar as possible a breakdown of the losses incurred. I also need to know exactly what happened when the business folded regarding premises and equipment. I am aware that you were left with significant debts and again details of the debts and how (if at all) these debts have been discharged would be most helpful.*

Ellie replies pointing out: (1) the debt of around £50,000 consisted of £38,000 owed to the bank with the remainder to other creditors (2) she had sent all the finance details in her possession, mainly the bank statements, and the contact details for the frail accountant to Mrs Archer two years before.

March 2002 Ellie to Mrs Archer:

> *It is now over two months since I heard from you. I would like to know if you received my letter of 23.1.02 and also confirmation you did in fact have all my husband's bank statements.*

How is the case proceeding and do you have any results after exchanging reports between the GP expert and the psychiatrist?

Ellie is right to be concerned. The accountant died about eighteen months ago, Carl's business accounts are due for shredding this month and we have no idea who holds them.

April 2002 Receiving no response, Ellie complains to the senior partner. She summarises the events since her last complaint culminating in the psychiatrist's report from which Mrs Archer concluded that a claim could not succeed. She continues:

Three months later I am still awaiting the outcome of Mrs Archer's proposals. I would like you to read my cousin's report because I believe Mrs Archer has ignored it, transfer our case to a colleague and obtain a consultant clinical psychologist's opinion.

Ellie was wrong to assume that Mrs Archer had ignored my commentary on the psychiatrist's report.

33

'*The purest treasure mortal times afford*
is spotless reputation'
— William Shakespeare, *Richard II*

Years later I'll read the file note Mrs Archer wrote on the day Ellie's letter arrived in her office:

> *Engaged reviewing the three page letter of the client and the twenty page "report" prepared by the client's cousin.*
>
> *The comments are not really of much assistance. They don't actually tackle the in depth issues in this case, merely go on about the peripheries such as interpretation of odd words [?TATT] and include scathing comments regarding the choice of expert and solicitor's conduct. Although she purportedly encloses her "CV" and suggests that she was an NHS consultant for 18 years, she does not actually list any of the hospitals where she has worked or what her position was in any of these hospitals.*

Ellie's comments could be rated as scathing; mine were analytical and I criticised the Medical Assistant's conduct. And how do you purportedly enclose something? You either enclose it or you don't. I actually, not purportedly, enclosed my extended research C.V. And in the first C.V. I'd sent them, I didn't *suggest* I was a consultant: I listed every hospital I'd ever worked in, with dates *and my position* in each. Two were well-known London teaching hospitals, and another two the hospitals where I had been *a consultant* – testimony to others' opinions of me. Mrs Archer continues:

Appended to the report is frankly bizarre and utterly unrelated newspaper clippings that I had to read through as they were part of the documentation sent to me by the client but frankly I fail to see the relevance of any of these and it just reconfirms my deep disquiet with this lady's involvement. She does not appear to appreciate the rigours of the Bolem test or to have an objective breakdown of the issues arising. The client however places total faith in Dr Payne who is her cousin [you've said that once] *and seems to be suggesting that I am on the 'side' of the psychiatrist and questions his independence.*

The relevance of the Appendix should have been obvious to a trained legal mind: my research on vascular risk factors was one useful piece in a large metabolic jigsaw whose political significance earned me recognition outside my profession and my country. The Bo*lam* (not, as these solicitors are apt to spell it, Bo*lem)* test is of liability whose rigours we expected the lawyers to explain. I *counted* the psychiatrist's errors and omissions and showed that all are prejudicial to the case.

I was the person her client's Litigation Friend turned to when devastated by her chosen expert's debatable claim that both had psychiatric histories going back many years. It needed medical knowledge to do this.

I've done it before, I'd do it again. I'd do it for my cousin, my best friend, or my worst enemy because I'd do it for the truth.

34

Between a rock and a hard place

Years later I'll read the responses of the two experts to each other's reports requested by Mrs Archer.

January 2002 Mrs Archer receives Dr Cooper's response to Dr Forrester's report. Her clear and cogent comments accord entirely with my criticisms. These stand out:

Specific comments

1. Dr Forrester: *...he presented to his GP in August 1990 with symptoms of poor concentration and memory coupled with some affective features of depression and anxiety...*

   Dr Cooper: *Anxiety is not generally considered to be an affective disorder* [psychiatric mood disorder]. *Depression is not recorded in the medical records in August 1990. There are no depressive features recorded such as (1) early morning waking (2) loss of appetite (3) loss of libido (4) depressed mood and affect (5) suicidal ideation. The absence of (1) and (5) are expressly documented. I do not understand what is meant by "affective features of depression".* The striking feature of the presentation in August 1990 is cognitive impairment but not depression.

2. Dr Forrester: …*TATT: which I understand to indicate an exaggerated presentation? totally above the top…*
Dr Cooper: *TATT is a common acronym found in medical records to denote "tired all the time".*

General comments and conclusion

Dr Cooper: *The copy of the report provided by my instructing solicitors consists of pages 1 to 12, and an unpaginated signed declaration. The report ends abruptly at the end of page 12 without a concluding section. I wonder if the copy provided is complete.* [Pages 13 – 15 of Dr Forrester's report were missing.]

He is a consultant psychiatrist and not a general medical practitioner; however, he provides an opinion on the standard of conduct of the general practitioner. His report purports to address the issues of causation, condition and prognosis. However, it considers matters relating to the "Bolam Principle" and the conduct of the general practitioner.

This case concerns the attribution of cognitive impairment to depression without even any attempt to assess such impairment or exclude organic causes. It is a fundamental and elementary principle of medicine that organic and physical causes of symptoms should be excluded before they are attributed to functional and psychogenic aetiologies. I consider that this represents the main failing of the general practitioner in August 1990.

I am instructed that "a conference may help to resolve some of these issues." I have addressed the main points of difference between my opinion and the psychiatrist's opinion. I do not consider that a conference would be helpful.

I confirm the opinion contained in my report dated 31 May 2001.

February 2002

Dr Forrester's response arrives in the solicitor's office.

It consists mainly of a recital of various claims made in his own report e.g. 'he had a history of depression from 1972…'

He addresses the 'TATT' issue thus:

> *I am grateful for your informing me that the abbreviation TATT stands for tired all the time. Knowing this, however, does not alter my views.*

…and concludes by stating his willingness to attend a conference.

Mrs Archer's dilemma may have been the reason for her failure to contact Ellie.

35

Back on the road

As we saw in Chapter 34, after no reply from Mrs Archer, Ellie complained to the senior partner in April.

May 2002
His reply with copy to me shows that he has carefully read and considered the issues, and discussed them with Mrs Archer.

Both accept that Mrs Archer made 'a fundamental error' in her suggestion that the claim cannot succeed simply because an earlier diagnosis would not have prevented or slowed the deterioration. There is a potential claim in that they would have been able to manage the financial affairs of the business had the diagnosis been made in 1990 leaving them with money in the bank instead of debts two years later.

My satisfaction with this delayed focus on the main issue is muted. In 1990, dementia was only one on the list of possibles (the differential diagnosis). The window of opportunity for a referral was between March and September *1991* when legislation was forcing them to re-plan the business and the GP should have been continuing to monitor Carl's cognitive difficulties.

It might or might not have been possible then to make a presumptive diagnosis of dementia with a high enough level of probability to tell the patient. But, with the knowledge that something was amiss without a cure just around the corner, they could have 'managed the financial affairs of the business …leaving them with money in the bank instead of debts.'

*

The senior partner agrees to transfer the day-to-day running of the case to an experienced personal injuries solicitor in the firm, Steve Glover, because Ellie's relationship with Mrs Archer 'has to some extent broken down.' He has sufficient concerns about Dr Forrester's report to justify obtaining the opinion of a consultant psychologist 'who has sufficient experience in dealing with clinical negligence claims'. What about experience in providing reports on this particular sub-speciality, I wonder. However, I know of two consultant psychologists who satisfy both these requirements.

Now the case is back on track I wonder about all the financial evidence which has been lost: not only is the accountant dead but Carl's business records probably went through a shredder a month ago. So although the senior partner has done his best to haul the case out of the morass I don't hold out much hope of success. The tone of a later paragraph in his letter suggests he doesn't either:

> *I have to say, however, that your case is by no means clear cut and even if a psychologist gives a favourable opinion, there are substantial hurdles to overcome before we obtain any or any significant compensation for you.*

Why wasn't Ellie warned of these substantial hurdles at the outset? Or didn't they exist then?

But the case is back on the road. To keep up the momentum I fax the solicitors the names and contact details of two consultant clinical psychologists. I know both have a good grasp of their subject and have provided medico-legal reports in dementia cases.

We wait. And wait. For months.

36

Eureka moments

They come years later when I read the senior partner's briefing to Steve Glover as he takes over the day-to-day handling of the case.

The senior partner points out that Caroline Archer's stance on the treatment of vascular risk factors does not exactly convey my position: I'd always very carefully stated in correspondence and discussions with him that a respected body of expert opinion believed that early treatment of vascular risk factors may slow down the rate of progress of vascular dementia. In one of her chronologies, Mrs Archer misconstrued my position thus:

> *The condition according to Dr Payne, a cousin of Mrs Valente, is treatable and if proper early diagnosis and treatment had been instigated he would have been in a better condition in any event.*

I never said that. Nor would I have. Everything fits now:

- Mrs Archer's focus on the late stages of dementia instead of on the time when legislation was forcing Carl to re-plan his business (March 1991 – September 1991)
- Her comment at our second meeting in January 2000 that my observations, on which she tacitly based her notion, were 'very helpful'.
- Her abruptly changed attitude to me at the meeting to

discuss Dr Cooper's report. She would have learned by
then that her notion was unsustainable.

- Her failure to deal with the financial information Ellie
  sent, contact the accountant before he died and obtain
  Carl's business records (Chapters 24, 34 and 35).

If only she'd said, when she should have done, something like:

> *So am I correct, doctor, in thinking that reducing his
> cholesterol/blood pressure/weight would have ameliorated
> the dementia?*

I would have disabused her of such an extravagant notion.

Dr Forrester's report

The senior partner's analysis, using Dr Cooper's and my comments,
makes these points (you will note my comments and italics):

- Dr Forrester 'appears to have misconstrued medical
  records to invent a pre-dementia psychiatric history in
  both the claimant and his wife' so appearing to have an
  unreasonable bias against the claimant.
- He 'definitely veers into the province of the GP expert
  and should not have done so. *By virtue of this he moves
  the breach of duty (want of care by GP) to May 1992.
  Crucially, this takes it to a point after the business had
  failed (March 1992)*'.

The business

The senior partner postulates that the sensible thing for Ellie to
have done when the accountant told her Carl's figures didn't make
sense was call in her son, a finance analyst. But why?

The accountant knew dependable Carl and his solvent
business like the back of his hand. (Absurd figures like £2,000,000

profits point not to a business problem but to a medical condition, e.g. bipolar disorder with inordinate optimism, or early dementia with impaired numeracy.) If their experienced long term GP couldn't solve it, how could a young finance analyst living two hundred miles away be expected to?

The response of their sons, both living some distance away, to Ellie's reports of the doctor telling Carl he was doing too much had always been: 'Dad's always been like that. You won't change him.' In those circumstances, it could have been a breach of family trust, confidentiality and loyalty of the sort that can split families. It was a step Ellie avoided taking until she felt impelled to in March 1992.

The senior partner considers tying the economic loss to the late diagnosis. He recalls a precedent: a case where wrong diagnosis of terminal cancer was held to have caused economic loss.

He doesn't know if the bank statements are adequate to support the claim but supposes that:

> *All we need is to show that it was reasonably in profit and that he had money in the bank in 1990. We are not trying to justify a continuing loss of earnings so we do not need to show that it would have continued to be profitable.*

That feels like a triumph of hope over experience.

Just as Carl's GP had failed to recognise the role of illness in his business demise, his lawyers failed to recognise the pivotal role of the 1991 legislation. There is no mention of it anywhere. Not in any of Ellie's statements, not in file notes, memos, letters, or phone calls, not in their instructions to experts or their reports, not in any of the fifteen kilograms of documents that the lawyers amassed in all the time they spent on the case.

37

'The truth, the whole truth, and nothing but the truth'

The senior partner continues in a somewhat different vein:

Vascular risk factors – he states (you will notice my italics: 'My concern is that *nobody* actually thinks that *any* treatment being given in 1990/91/92 actually did *any good at all'* – a point made by Dr Forrester.

A point made in a report containing errors, omissions and debatable points by a psychiatrist with no declared interest in dementia. Dementia is a syndrome with both genetic and environmental risk factors, including vascular, which can be managed with potential benefit. It is nicely summarised by McCullagh, Craig, McIlroy and Passmore in their review article (published around the time of Dr Forrester's report) on dementia risk factors:[43]

> *In contrast to the advances made in our understanding of genetic risk factors in Alzheimer's disease, identification of non-genetic or environmental risk factors has been slower. Non-inherited risk factors are likely to be important, as monozygotic* [identical] *twin concordance rates (for Alzheimer type dementia) reach only 40%* [reference given].[44] *Different ethnic groups living in similar environments show comparable prevalence rates* [for Alzheimer type dementia], *again suggesting a role*

for environmental factors. Studies, which are often beset with methodological problems, have produced repeatedly conflicting results...Apolipoprotein E status [genetic] in particular appears to modulate the influence of several environmental risk factors.'

The senior partner continues:

...the question that can and must be answered by reference to current knowledge *i.e. what do doctors now think of the treatment that was given then – I suspect not very much. ...there is a letter from the GP expert giving her comments on whether or not treatment would have done any good even if he had been correctly diagnosed: answer, no.*

'Answer, no' is based, not on a report from a specialist in dementia or vascular disorders, but on a comment in a GP's letter of which we knew nothing. Her view that 'the evidence for the supposed treatment of dementia is unconvincing' does acknowledge that it exists which is more than can be said for Dr Forrester, the specialist.

I assume that the evidence Dr Cooper is dissenting from is this: expert reviews in mainstream journals like the UK's *Lancet*[45] and *British Medical Journal*[46] the latter by two specialists in a memory clinic:

...evidence exists that controlling vascular risk factors such as hypertension [high blood pressure] and diabetes and using an anti-platelet drug can improve cognitive functioning...vascular risk factors such as hypertension, diabetes, and hypercholesterolaemia [raised cholesterol] can by themselves cause cognitive impairment. This led some

investigators to advocate identifying and treating those risk
factors regardless of the cause of dementia, especially with
reports of an association between vascular risk factors and
Alzheimer's disease.

Secondly, the view of three other UK experts (Harvey, Fox and Rossor) in their *1999 Dementia Handbook*[47] for medical and other health care workers:

In the introduction:

...the course of vascular dementia may be modified by
active intervention aimed at underlying risk factors...
effective and specific support can only be delivered to
patients and caregivers if a name has been put to their
disease.

On vascular dementia:

...Eliciting the presence of vascular risk factors, such as
hypertension, *smoking, cardiovascular disease, diabetes*
and hypercholesterolaemia [raised cholesterol] *are*
important, particularly since managing these risk factors
may reduce the rate of progression of the disease.

That's all I ever said so why didn't they listen?

The importance of treating vascular risk factors in dementia (primarily for the prevention of strokes) had become a matter for public guidance in the US by *1992* (Gruetzner, *Alzheimer's A Caregiver's Guide and Sourcebook).*[48] And in *1999 (this was 2002)* I had even found a well-used copy for Ellie in the WITHDRAWN FOR SALE section of our small branch library.

Yet the senior partner disdained the accumulating evidence

of internationally recognised experts that correcting vascular risk factors may slow the decline in intellectual function.

The senior partner's memo to Steve Glover states:

> *The attached chronology which has been put together by Caroline* perfectly and reasonably accurately *summarises the position in the case.*

I turn to Mrs Archer's chronology, and concentrate on the more significant errors. She dismisses Carl's debts as 'pure economic loss', failing to acknowledge the parallel with the senior partner's quoted case of economic loss held to be caused by a wrong diagnosis. *I don't believe it.* She has no more supporting evidence for her current stance (correct or incorrect) than when she took the case on – because she made no attempt to acquire it. She states:

> *When the business finally collapsed in March 1992 it was clearly in a very difficult state already as there had been problems with bookkeeping for* a couple of years at least [i.e. from *March 1990* or before].

No! The bank statements, all we have to go on, show that the business was solvent until July 1991, and £5000 in debt by September 1991. *The problems with bookkeeping before then were inside Carl's head not his business.* The evidence on the business itself may not have stood up to forensic scrutiny but *that's what we went to the lawyers to find out.*

As we saw earlier, Mrs Archer took a quick look at the bank statements in 2000, dismissed them as uninformative and decided to come back to them when she had time which it seems she never had.

Mrs Archer concludes:

I do think the way forward with this case is a conference with the attendance of Dr Forrester. I do not think the attendance of Dr Cooper is necessary. I have not revisited the extensive comments of Dr Payne who is a relation. I would suggest her remarks are put to Counsel wholesale for Counsel's consideration and Dr Forrester should be forewarned and sent a complete set of enclosures from Dr Payne that Counsel has received.'

I don't know what she hopes to achieve.

So Steve Glover would have been working from Mrs Archer's chronology and opinions that weren't in accordance with those of the senior partner despite his expressed belief in their 'perfect and reasonable' accuracy.

The senior partner ends with a suggestion that any instructions are cleared with and agreed by Dr Payne – 'simply to avoid any further criticism'.

38

An odd incident

Summer 2002

I'd made an arrangement to visit my elderly mother who lives in the same town as Ellie. When I give her a ring before I set off, she says her GP is calling to do his monthly visit but we'll be back by then from lunch at our usual cafe.

She's been with that GP for a long time and she thinks the world of him. Always gives him some of the strawberries from our garden that we take her each year. Occasionally I've phoned him when I've been concerned about her. I've always had every confidence in him and more than once been grateful when he's gone beyond the basic call of duty. Sometimes I've accompanied her into the surgery and he's not had a problem with it. We count ourselves very lucky.

We've been back from lunch for about half an hour when Mum sees his car pull up outside. When I open the door to let him in, he looks aghast.

'What are you doing here?' he asks. I'm gobsmacked. It feels like an accusation from someone who's been betrayed.

He asks: 'Did you know I was coming?'

I manage to get the word 'Yes' out of my mouth.

Muttering something like 'what's it all about' he goes in to see Mum. He deals with her general health and medication, then asks about her feet and legs. She'd been troubled recently by pins-and-needles. He goes into it some more then asks me if there's anything

I want to add. I mention a possibility. He's done the blood tests to exclude it but the results aren't back yet. In one leap he's across the room to Mum's phone and getting them from the Path Lab.

Everything's normal as expected. End of consultation. I see him to the door. He gives me an intent look.

'I don't know what's behind all this,' he tells me. Again I sense that he feels betrayed.

The feeling's mutual because I know that if I'd ever for one moment had any doubts about his treatment of my mother he's the kind of person I could have discussed things with face-to-face. I'd never have gone behind his back.

My intuition says it's connected with the case. There are professional, social, cultural and business ties between the towns: Ellie's and Mum's, the solicitor's, and mine.

After Mum dies about nine months later I send him a handwritten note of thanks telling him how much I'd appreciated never having to worry at any time about the standard of care she received from him, and being able to get in touch with him whenever I was concerned about her.

Although I receive a cordial handwritten reply, the feeling will always remain, I suspect for both of us, that the incident has tarnished a once rewarding relationship.

I breathe a sigh of relief that I'm retired because it feels as if the twelve-bore shotgun's been fired again.

39

'I just want the truth'

September 2002

One of the psychologists I suggested to the solicitors feels he can help with the case. He explains his particular expertise in dementia diagnosis and the extent of his medico-legal experience, whilst pointing out that it didn't include a court appearance.

Mr Glover writes to Ellie saying that although he appreciates 'the interest your cousin is taking in this matter' they would prefer to drop him because: he has moved further away (to about the same distance as the other experts); he has never given evidence in Court; the solicitors don't know him. He asks Ellie to consider her position. He reminds her that the claim is publicly funded. If the psychologist provides 'a report that does not assist, the Legal Services Commission would not be prepared to meet the cost of another report, although that is not to suggest that the report will be unhelpful, merely to advise her of the position.'

Ellie says she has no problems with that. It's the truth she's after.

His report, finished just before Christmas, reaches the solicitors on 2nd January 2003.

40

'The truth untold'
— Wilfred Owen, *Strange Meeting*, 1917

Dr Miller's fourteen page report is in standard medico-legal format.

He begins by listing his qualifications, research and experience: First Class Honours degree and PhD in Psychology; papers on clinical psychology (mainly measurement and management of cognitive dysfunction including dementia); over ten years' experience in medico-legal work including a course on the 'Woolf Report'; [49,50] membership of professional bodies; university lectureships and his current post of Consultant Neuropsychologist giving all commencement and termination dates.

He lists the materials relied on: medical records; solicitors' chronology; Ellie's statement; Dr Cooper's report and correspondence; the solicitors' instructions, one of which crucially does not accurately reflect Ellie's contention. It reads:

If a treatment/referral had been made in August 1990, what would the likely diagnosis have been and, in particular, what information or advice would have been given to Mr Valente and/or Mrs Valente with regard to his capacity to manage his own affairs?

As we saw in Chapter 12, the case hinges on what information should have been given to the couple with regard to Carl's capacity to manage his own affairs, not in August 1990, but sometime between 25th March 1991 and 25th September 1991.

Dr Miller, writing in an academic and somewhat discursive style (indicative of an expert who's still enthused by his chosen subject), notes:

1. The rapid onset of cognitive defects could have been due to a brain tumour or a series of strokes.
2. Stress responses and depression can cause severe cognitive impairment but his report shows that this diagnostic conundrum is solvable.
3. The external evidence that the accountant was, for the first time in years, having difficulty understanding Carl's figures supports the contention that cognitive defects would have shown on psychological tests. And, although it came from Ellie, it could be verified. [Little does he know, I'll think years later, that the opportunity to verify the external evidence had already been lost with (a) the death of the accountant (b) the probable shredding of the business documents.]
4. Ellie's statement is 'unfortunately undated'.
5. The effect of Ellie's visit to the GP in March 1991 about Carl was his prescription − for her − of a two week course of a tranquilliser.

His opinions and conclusions are best summarised in his own words:

Overall, it is not possible to state whether Mr Valente was suffering from dementia in 1990.

He continues:

That [the diagnosis] *would only have been possible if we had results from various tests. There is* prima facie *evidence of cognitive deterioration though. These were errors which*

153

were being made as well as the loss of a well-learned skill – bookkeeping which would implicate working memory. These are highly suggestive of organicity [he means neurological rather than psychiatric or stress] *and should have been followed up by a cognitive assessment. It is unacceptable that formal assessment was only carried out 5 years after the initial complaint despite that complaint being repeated* [he is referring to the tests in 1995 – when Carl was told to stop driving, leaving Ellie wondering how much sooner it could have been picked up].

Given the nature of the deficits present and the likelihood that tests available at that time would have indicated such deficits [he made that point elsewhere in his report] it would have been important to have advised both Mr and Mrs Valente of those deficits...*Certainly, if there was poor performance on what were known as 'frontal lobe' tests* [to be expected, he notes, because of Carl's difficulty with accounts and decision making; he notes too that the CT scan performed eventually showed frontal lobe atrophy] then the clinician would be obliged to inform the client of this as well as to discuss the consequences of the results for everyday practice.

So a consultant neuropsychologist's opinion is that something significant was happening inside Carl's head – probably not diagnostic of dementia in 1990 – which the couple should have been told about because of its impact on their everyday lives.

For me, his report said all that was needed. But not for the lawyers as we would discover years later.

41

Res ipsa loquitur
The facts speak for themselves

Years later we discover what happened between Mr Glover apparently taking over the case in May 2002 and receiving Dr Miller's report in January 2003.

May 2002
Mr Glover discovers that neither of the two psychologists I suggested is known to the organisation which, according to Mrs Archer, runs the country's most authoritative database of experts specialising in clinical negligence. It's the one that threw up Dr Forrester's name.

The absence of this credential doesn't trouble me: a spokeswoman for the organisation confirmed my suspicions that they did little vetting. All you had to do to get your name on their books/data base was give them your contact details plus whatever information you chose about your area of expertise.

Mr Glover plans to ask Dr Cooper whether, had Dr Bromwich carried out some simple cognitive tests, these would have justified a referral to a psychologist in August 1990. Then see whether the psychologist will confirm that a referral then would have led to a diagnosis of dementia.

It's an irrelevant hypothetical question. In August 1990 there were three main conditions for the GP to consider (the differential diagnosis): dementia, depression and too high an alcohol consumption. It was between 25th March 1991 when

Ellie saw Dr Bromich about Carl and 25th September 1991, when Carl saw the doctor himself, when he should have been referred to a specialist, whether or not any 'simple cognitive tests' had been done – because Carl wasn't getting better and needed immediate thorough investigation.

June 2002

Mr Glover then considers the bank statements noting that the business was permanently in overdraft from July 1991 and, in fact, had been overdrawn before then. And that when the business finally collapsed in March 1992 it was 'clearly in a very difficult state already as there had been problems with bookkeeping for a couple of years at least'. These deliberations owe more to the solicitors' inaccurate chronology than they do to the truth contained in the bank statements. To be fair, Mr Glover may have been hampered by the senior partner's rating of the chronology as 'perfectly and reasonably accurate'.

I've had enough of this. I'll demonstrate the truth, with no mistakes, in the way I know best. I find some sheets of graph paper from my pre-retirement days and get started.

With one small square representing one day on the horizontal axis and one small square representing £1000 on the vertical axis, I plot a graph of the bank statements. It takes a long time because I do it twice to correct any errors, and again to make sure all errors have been eliminated. Then I add vertical arrows pointing downwards from the top to indicate important events on the exact day when they happened: doctor's visits; the 1991 legislation; closure of the account; repayment of debts etc.

These facts stand out:

1. Between 4th January 1991 (when the bank statements start) and 9th July 1991, Carl kept the account in balance between zero and £12,000 topping up within one

day on the odd occasions when it dipped into the red by up to £2000. Carl's pencilled annotations were on every transaction. There is no evidence for Mrs Archer's assertion that when the business finally collapsed in March 1992 'it was clearly in a very difficult state already as there had been problems with bookkeeping for a couple of years *at least.*'

2. On 9 July 1991, within the crucial time window March 25 (Ellie's visit to Dr Bromwich about Carl) to September 25 1991 (Carl's visit to Dr Bromwich complaining of being tired all the time), the account went into the red by £5000 and stayed there. *This is (a) when the GP should have referred Carl for investigation (b) when legislation forced them to make a decision about the business.*

3. In September 1991, Carl stopped annotating the transactions: his brain had given up. The debts to the bank escalated until, by March 1992, they had reached £38,000.

So the business was solvent until July 1991 by which time the referral could have been made, and in debt by £5000 in September 1991 by which time the referral should have been made.

July 2002

The next day Mr Glover writes to the organisation which recommended Dr Forrester because Ellie had complained to them about his report. In it he refers to me as a retired *psychologist.*

Psychologists have degrees in psychology, not medicine (although some are dual qualified). Theirs is a diagnostic and non-medical therapies speciality. Psychiatrists have degrees in medicine and a postgraduate qualification in psychiatry.

I have a first degree in medicine, not psychology. I have a postgraduate qualification, experience at consultant level and research in a scientific branch of medicine relevant to this case. My field of particular expertise within my speciality (cholesterol and triglyceride abnormalities, atherosclerosis, vascular pathology, and the biochemical basis of the dementias and their management) means that I had a better understanding than anyone else involved so far of the pathology underlying the relevant conditions.

January 2003

Mr Glover sends Dr Miller's report to Mrs Archer for her observations on the day it was received in the office. Having 'read through this carefully', she emails him later that day. In the half hour she spent, she seems to have had difficulty with finding useful criticisms as these examples show:

1. *It is not for the psychologist to criticise the GP's conduct. We have to rely on the GP expert for that...*

Fair enough but it does not sit well with her later criticism of the psychologist for failing to 'address the Bolam test ie what would a reasonable GP have done'. That, too, is for the GP expert, not the psychologist, to answer. And Dr Cooper has already answered it.

2. She notes the psychologist's reference to 'client' (Carl) instead of 'clients' (Carl and Ellie).

I had dismissed it as a 'typo' (for checking later) because his intended meaning of 'clients' (the couple) was clear from the previous sentence.

3. She notes that the psychologist has 'comprehensively failed to answer question 2' which is: *Express an opinion as to whether if a referral to a psychologist had been made in August 1990 what would the likely outcome in terms of limiting and/or controlling the disease/condition have been.*

The long-term outcome of *medical* management is outside a psychologist's field of specialist expertise to give an opinion on although, as a consultant neuropsychologist, he would have the necessary working knowledge of it.

Res ipsa loquitur. The facts speak for themselves.

42

'I was there'

Mr Glover arranges a conference between himself, the barrister (Miss Sawyer), the psychologist (Dr Miller), Ellie, and me – after asking Ellie whether she wishes her cousin to be present. So I'll hear what goes on if nothing else.

At our pre-meeting with Mr Glover, Ellie and I are given a copy of Miss Sawyer's Preparation for Conference notes. It's clear and authoritative consisting of relevant legal points and what Miss Sawyer sees as the weaknesses of the case – what I'd hoped we'd get from the solicitors.

Miss Sawyer begins by going through the preparation notes. Looking directly at me, she explains that if someone's cancer isn't diagnosed until it's too late to enjoy what's left of his life, he may have a claim for a missed 'once in a lifetime holiday'. I wonder if she's implying that, by contrast, if your dementia isn't diagnosed until you're too far gone to enjoy anything, you won't get anything. I open my mouth to speak but her eyes flick away.

In her discussions with Dr Miller, these points emerge:

1. Dementia was one of the differential diagnoses the GP should have had in mind; the case becomes stronger by 1991 rather than 1990.
2. In a man of fifty-three, Dr Miller wouldn't think depression, he would think organic, meaning neurological

rather than psychological e.g. brain tumour.

3. Dr Miller says that, on the balance of probabilities, with *a referral in 1991* they would have found an executive function defect [frontal lobe problem causing difficulty with figures, reasoning, planning, problem solving] and would have diagnosed dementia. That would have given them time to do something about the business.

During this discussion, a puzzling exchange occurs. In an uncharacteristically dogmatic gesture, Dr Miller jabs the page in front of him with his forefinger, turns to me and says: '*That* is a psychiatric history.' He's referring to Carl's psychiatric history prior to the onset of dementia – non-existent according to Carl's own doctors. I dismiss as incredible the thought that he could be defending the opinions of a colleague in a related speciality. But I feel uneasy.

Years later, I will find that my incredible idea may have been near the mark. The detailed chronology used by the barrister includes relevant extracts from Carl's and Ellie's GP notes. But crucial sections are not extracts of the original notes: they are *verbatim copies of Dr Forrester's mistranscriptions and omissions appearing to show that six physical complaints of Carl's, from minor to serious, were psychiatric.* If this was the chronology Dr Miller had been working from, it would entirely explain his belief that Carl had a previous psychiatric history.

The barrister's chronology also records the result of a cholesterol test that attracted a much different consultant comment from that on Carl's first visit to the GP in 1990 which is not included. Hardly surprising as it was done in *1998* when Carl was about to go into full-time care. What its purpose was I cannot imagine. Certainly it bears little relationship to Carl's metabolic state until 1990–1991.

*

161

Miss Sawyer asks Ellie why she, a business person herself, didn't intervene sooner in his business activities to prevent the debts. Ellie says that she'd never interfered in her husband's business before and didn't feel she should do so then. Miss Sawyer thanks Ellie for being honest – and shoots me a look. My eyes don't fall but I feel very uneasy now.

A better answer to the question would have been that having seen the doctor herself about Carl's mental state, Ellie believed that he, a doctor, would deal with it so at the time she didn't feel she should interfere in Carl's business.

The meeting ends with Dr Miller agreeing to provide the name and contact details of a local neurologist with a particular interest in dementia. Although I'm sure that, if the case is winnable, this capable and helpful barrister will win it, my intuition says it won't happen.

Years later, I read Mr Glover's pre-conference notes:

Phone call to Counsel

1. *The solicitors have reservations about engaging Dr Miller as an expert because he has 'no medico-legal experience'.* That isn't quite what Dr Miller said. He explained that he had ten years' experience of writing expert reports and had attended a course on the Woolf reforms[49,50] but had never given expert evidence in court.

2. *Mr Glover tells Miss Sawyer that I complained twice.* No, I did not. Ellie complained twice off her own bat, the second time enclosing supporting documents which I had prepared for her.

Instructions to Counsel

1. Mr Glover has revised his description of me from retired psychologist to registered medical practitioner.

2. His wording suggests that he checked with the

General Medical Council despite more detailed information on me being available in his own files.

3. *Counsel will further note that Dr Payne, on behalf of the Litigation Friend* [Ellie acting for Carl who can't speak for himself], *has twice registered complaints.* How many more times? Ellie complained twice off her own bat.

4. *It appears that the claimant is mainly concerned to recover his business losses…The solicitors have not, to date, instructed forensic accountants to review the appropriate business accounts, mindful that the claim is publicly funded.* And mindful that *the accounts probably no longer exist?*

5. The claimant set up a 'disastrous business venture' in 1991. *What?* Carl was forced – by 1991 *legislation* – to draw in his business horns when he was becoming incapable of setting up anything, even curtain rails.

6. *The claimant's son is a leading business analyst who appears to live with the Litigation Friend so he might reasonably have been expected to notice his father's deteriorating condition and perhaps have taken steps to intervene. What?* Either he lived with the Litigation Friend or he didn't. He didn't. He lived about two hundred miles away. Fact. And I ponder again on how a young finance analyst, whether he lives in Bognor Regis or Wolverhampton and however close his relationship to the patient, might *reasonably* have been expected to notice a medical condition that an experienced GP couldn't see right under his nose.

No wonder I felt uneasy in Conference.

43

'I told you I was ill'

– Spike Milligan 1918–2002

Years later I read all the documentation for the period after the conference with the barrister in March 2003 to the end of the case in September 2003.

As agreed, Dr Miller gives the solicitors the name of a local neurologist specialising in dementia. After discussing the case with Mrs Archer, Mr Glover concludes that the instruction should be to a psychiatrist. Mrs Archer next suggests a psychologist she knows based in another town an inconvenient drive away.

Another psychologist – from whom Mr Glover requests a report, again describing Carl's business downsize as a 'disastrous business venture'.

This psychologist recommends obtaining a report from a neurologist specialising in dementia based in the same town. Mr Glover requests an opinion from him, yet again describing Carl's business downsize as a 'disastrous business venture'.

I have a flashback to the Complaints Manager's description of the couple's established businesses as 'business ventures' (Chapter 15).

In mid-August, Ellie receives a letter from Mr Glover enclosing the neurologist's report. She sends me a copy.

Mr Glover's letter to Ellie
He begins by asking her to concentrate on the 'Discussion and

opinion' section and to ignore 'the odd little typographical error' which is 'not surprising in such a long report'. I decode the lawyer-speak: 'We don't want your cousin going through this report with her nit-comb'.

The letter continues:

The neurologist has set out the differential diagnoses that were possible…he points out that many earlier diagnoses of dementia prove to be false…the implication is that a cautious approach has to be taken to avoid an early, maybe wrong, diagnosis of dementia.

Quite so. But doing nothing about worsening cognitive defects in a businessman in his early fifties constitutes a careless, not a cautious, approach.

The neurologist raises the question of what advice *should be given to a patient with* mild to moderate depression *and he suggests that an opinion from the GP expert should be obtained in this respect. I am not at all sure that this is necessary, or that I can justify this further expenditure to the Legal Services Commission, and the neurologist himself, in my view, practically says as much in the last sentence of that paragraph.*

Agreed – because the real question is this: what *information* (not advice) should be given to a patient with *significant cognitive defects* (not mild to moderate depression).

Simply put, if one of the diagnoses was mild to moderate depression *I cannot see that as a result any GP would reasonably have told your husband to close down or alternatively not to start up a business. From your own experience do you not agree?*

I agree because people see doctors for information about their illness -whether it's depression, Sjögren's syndrome, renal colic or dementia – not for advice about their business.

> *Importantly, the neurologist does suggest that even in a specialist centre with a complete clinical assessment the probability of an accurate diagnosis of* dementia [he's switched here from depression to dementia] *at that point would have been no more than 27%. It seems to me, therefore, that if Mr Valente's GP had, at that point in time advised Mr Valente to cease any business activity then this advice would, on a 3:1 basis, have been incorrect/ inappropriate.*

Agreed, whatever the odds ratio, because people see doctors about their illness not their business.

> *I would be pleased to hear from you with any comments that you may have but I am afraid I do have to make it clear that I cannot see that the Legal Services Commission can be persuaded to fund this matter further.*

The neurologist's report
He explains that he is a practising neurologist with a particular interest in disturbances of higher mental function and memory, citing his research publications in peer-reviewed journals. He lists the supporting documents sent by the solicitors. Dr Forrester's and Dr Miller's reports aren't listed.

Ignoring the typos (the report looks as if it's been typed from a dictation tape), I note these items:

1. He thinks *some of the entries are out of sequence* in Carl's GP notes, thereby joining the ranks of the experts on this case perplexed about dates.

2. Referring to Carl's first visit, he states that the GP identified a 'somatic (bodily) sign of depression i.e. difficulty with getting a refreshing sleep'.

It is not a specific sign of depression. Dr Cooper's comment on the same visit is that there were no signs specific to depression e.g. no early waking and, explicitly, no suicidal ideation.

3. The neurologist seems not to have noticed the GP's note to 'See husband' after Ellie saw him about Carl in March 1991 – it does not appear in his otherwise verbatim quote of the visit.

The neurologist's other interesting points are:

4. *Dementia is the term given to the group of clinical conditions in which there is a progressive decline in two or more specified cognitive functions, one of which must be memory, persistent over a period of six months. Generally but not necessarily it starts with a decline in memory. The defects must be sufficiently severe to cause impairment in occupational or social functioning.*

This fitted Carl by 25th March 1991, the date of Ellie's visit to the GP about him when the business was still solvent.

5. *The diagnosis is clinical, supported by investigations including formal psychological tests, which in the early stages may be normal or near normal. Investigations exclude brain tumours and metabolic disease such as hypothyroidism* [under-active thyroid] *and vitamin B12* [the pernicious anaemia vitamin] *deficiency.* In the younger person ie below fifty-five years of age more extensive investigations are required.

6. *Extrapolating backwards from Carl's later mental state screening tests, the tests would have been normal if done in 1990.*

The neurologist does not extrapolate backwards to *1991* when the referral should have been made.

7. *Mr Valente's symptoms in 1990 were probably the start of his Alzheimer's dementia, and the report of making mistakes at work should have alerted the GP to further enquiry from Mr Valente's wife about the nature of his difficulties. There may be issues of confidentiality if Mr Valente did not agree to this however.*

The GP's declared intention (as we have seen, not noted by the neurologist) to 'See husband' after Ellie's visit on March 1991 indicates that he'd decided he would have to deal with the confidentiality issue. It's a familiar problem for family doctors for which the General Medical Council has helpful guidelines. We'll never know why the GP failed to act on his intention.

I have a flashback to this sentence in Dr Forrester's report:

It is conceivable that a referral in 1991 may have resulted in the identification of a very early dementing process and then it would have been theoretically possible for Mr Valente and his family to negotiate the business problems at an earlier stage.

and to this paragraph in Dr Miller's report:

…There is prima facie *evidence of cognitive deterioration though. There were errors which were being made as well as the loss of a well-learned skill* (bookkeeping which would implicate working memory). *Given the nature of*

*the deficits present and the likelihood that tests available
at that time would have indicated such deficits* it would
have been important to have advised them both of those
deficits...*Certainly, if there was poor performance on
what were known as 'frontal lobe' tests then the clinician
would be obliged to inform the client* [a probable 'typo': it
should have read clients] *of this as well as to discuss the
consequences of the results for everyday practice.'*

The experts are agreed that Carl's symptoms in 1990–1991 were
the start of his dementia and the GP should have investigated
further given Carl's age, their nature and the trouble they were
causing.

*Only Dr Miller explicitly recognises the obligation of the clinician
to explain to the couple the implications of the cognitive deficits
themselves for everyday living. He alone has gone over the top into
the communications No Man's Land which divides clinicians from
their patients, their colleagues and other professionals, sometimes with
catastrophic results.*

So, although there wasn't a definitive/definite/precise
diagnosis – call it what you will – there were cognitive deficits
which should have been explained to Carl and Ellie. As if the
mechanic, having got advice from the main agent, knows there's
a fault somewhere in your car's engine management system that
they'll have to keep an eye on, and tells you to be careful how you
drive the car until it's sorted.

A fortnight later – and thirteen years to the day after he first went
to his GP complaining of what would eventually be diagnosed as
a vascular dementia – Giancarlo Valente dies aged sixty-six.

44

Bastards: nailed?

The day after Carl's funeral, Ellie answers Mr Glover's letter apologising for not having responded sooner. She says she would have welcomed Dr Cooper's opinion as the neurologist suggested but she feels any comment on the neurologist's report would be futile.

Motivated perhaps by sympathy plus a desire to get rid of the case once and for all, Mr Glover writes to Dr Cooper enclosing a copy of the neurologist's report. He receives a prompt reply:

> *...The neurologist has recommended that an opinion is obtained from myself about the normal advice given by general practitioners to patients with mild/moderate* depression *about life decisions.*
>
> *I am instructed to consider whether* in those circumstances [depression presumably] *a general practitioner would have advised a patient with a business background to dispose urgently of his business.*
>
> *This is not a matter on which I am able to advise. It is not usual for general practitioners to give business advice to their patients...*

Mr Glover writes to Ellie:

> *...I am sure you will appreciate Dr Cooper's prompt reply. Unfortunately, I cannot see that it actually assists with the*

170

claim. On the face of it therefore I really cannot advise the Legal Services Commission to extend the Legal Aid Certificate…I am sorry that we here and the barrister have not been able to achieve the result that you had hoped for.

We are left alone. I'm feeling useless, demeaned and frustrated.

My last involvement in a medico-legal case and this is how it's ended. In all the reports I've done (not many by some experts' standards, but a fair few) the outcome has always been according to my conclusion, irrespective of whether it was favourable to the party that engaged me.

I can't have put things in the right way, I think. I said too much. I said too little. I spoke too soon. I spoke too late.

I've let Ellie down.

She phones a fortnight later. She's joining her son and his family on their ski holiday after Christmas and is off to buy a ski outfit that will make her look like Princess Diana. We laugh at the impossibility. Then she says: 'A clinical negligence solicitor's just set up in town.'

'Oh,' I say without enthusiasm.

'I'm going to see him about whether it's worth having another go at the claim. I'd like you to come with me.'

Huh, I think, I wasn't much use last time. But she trusts me and she's honouring her promise to Carl. So we see him together. Once he has considered all the first solicitor's documents and my written comments on the case, he will give Ellie his opinion.

A few weeks later he sends Ellie his clear and dispassionate observations on the strengths and weaknesses of a potential claim, describing my notes as helpful. Dare I feel encouraged, I wonder? This is how it looks (my italics and you'll note my comments):

1. The basis of the claim: if the diagnosis of dementia had been made *or the risk of it recognised when it should have been*, the advice received would have enabled them

to make lifestyle changes, particularly regarding the business, thus avoiding much distress and financial loss. Damages claimed would be in respect of pain and suffering and financial loss suffered before the formal diagnosis in 1993.

2. Conference with Counsel:

   (a) *there appears to be no formal barrister's opinion* [I hadn't spotted that]

   (b) the barrister's concern that the psychologist may not prove to be a good witness in court

3. Liability: the prospects of establishing that the GP's standard of care was unacceptable appear to be good. Outcome in the event of establishing liability – picture less certain:

   (a) views of the three specialists (psychiatrist, psychologist and neurologist) appear to differ in ways the court may not find acceptable.

   (b) the business losses would be the major element in any award but he has seen *no evidence whatsoever* on the financial state of the business and it could become a contentious issue calling for the evidence of forensic accountants [no surprises there].

4. Funding (from Carl's estate):

   (a) The recoverable damages must be likely to outstrip the costs incurred, otherwise the claim becomes uneconomic, *however important the issues involved.*

   (b) Ellie could proceed as a privately funded litigant or by persuading a solicitor to act on a conditional fee agreement basis, a.k.a. 'no win, no fee.' The disadvantage is that if she loses she would be liable for the defence costs.

   (c) At this stage he could not commit himself to

acting on a conditional fee agreement basis: he
would need to obtain more information from
the experts, particularly the GP and the neurologist, before forming a view [he hasn't ruled it
out so he must think the case might have some
merit].

5. There is a time limit of three years from the date of
Carl's death.

Ellie is in a catch-22. Almost certainly none of Carl's business
records exist. She either does nothing, failing to honour her
promise to Carl, or she risks losing all of Carl's estate, everything
they'd ever worked for, in an unsung and futile attempt to keep
that promise.

In the end she decides not to proceed and pays the solicitor
his substantial but well-earned fee thereby becoming the owner of
a box containing about fifteen kilograms of documents. She puts
it away in a cupboard because she can't bear either to go through it
or to throw everything out.

A few years later, a chance remark at an Alzheimer's Society
meeting brings all the unhappy memories flooding back. She talks
to a friend who happens to be a trained counsellor.

'Ellie,' she says, 'you've carried that burden long enough.
Drop it. Burn everything.'

She tells me this the day before we are due to meet at a family
funeral. I say: 'Yes, you've carried that burden long enough but
please don't do that. I'll take it from you.'

I put the box in a corner of the study when I get home. Many
times over the next four years, I would take the lid off, then put it
back, curbed by forebodings of what it contained.

One morning I'm listening to a radio programme on the
suffering caused by late diagnosis of dementia. I hear Carl's words
of years ago: 'Nail the bastards.' And the words of victims of
medical mishaps: 'I don't want this to happen to anyone else.'

I open it and this time I don't put the lid back on until I've trawled through everything.

That's how I discovered what was and wasn't in the first solicitors' memos, emails, file notes and letters, and the answers to three questions. Why wasn't Ellie given similar advice to the second solicitor's at the outset? Why wasn't all the evidence of Carl's business finances obtained before it was too late when the business losses were the major element of the case? Why did the first solicitors view the long-term clinical consequences of incorrect treatment as the major element when their client did not? That's how we nailed the bastards.

PART 4

On Reflection

'And the truth shall make you free.'

– John 8, 32

45

'If that's justice, then I'm a banana'
— Ian Hislop, editor, *Private Eye*

Four years of legal process led nowhere. Carl and Ellie, like the majority of clinical negligence claimants, ended up with nothing.

The case seemed to start well enough. At our first meeting I sensed Mrs Archer was moved by the sight of her client, silent immobile Carl, and his wife, Ellie, who had become his mother.

An idea forms in my mind.

Mrs Archer already had a good track record in a difficult legal speciality. I can imagine how youthful enthusiasm made her determined to pull off a rewarding landmark victory. Perhaps she reasoned that a claim for personal injury caused by clinical negligence would stand more chance of success than one based on economic loss caused by the missed diagnosis. She certainly seems to have taken only a passing interest in the financial side.

But the economic loss, Ellie's main concern, was more readily quantifiable than the personal injury and capable of accurate correlation with the time when Carl should have been referred for specialist investigation. I'd always envisaged that the lawyers would tag any personal injury award to the pecuniary damage settlement.

Enter Mrs Baker. She would have qualified in nursing when training was didactic, dementia syndromes were viewed, certainly by non-specialists, as a single untreatable degenerative disease, and high cholesterol levels had no connection whatsoever with any manifestation of atherosclerosis, not even heart attacks. Her likely mindset would have been: 'You can't treat dementia so it's kinder to say nothing. The doctors did the right thing. End of.'

Mrs Baker may well have been concerned by the direction in which the case was heading, and the amount of taxpayers' money being spent on it. As the Medical Assistant, she may have asked around about 'whether lowering your cholesterol cures dementia' and been firmly told: 'No!'

Mrs Archer seemed to be working from home at times when the work of the firm's clinical negligence department had increased so much that another solicitor (Mrs Carter) was brought in to help during the case.

Had Dr Cooper, the GP expert, concluded that Carl's GP's management was not negligent, the case would have ended there. But, clearly and unequivocally, she didn't. Mrs Archer was stuck with pursuing a an unsustainable personal injury claim. It would have become expedient to drop the case. The opportunity came with Dr Forrester's report but, as we have seen, it actually succeeded in prolonging its life for a couple of years.

So what happened to Mrs Archer's early enthusiasm? Perhaps I'd misread the vibes. But that begs the question of why she ever took the case on at all: she could reasonably have used the argument that an application for Legal Aid must demonstrate that the likely award will exceed the expenditure in a ratio of four (or it might then have been six) to one as a reason for not taking on the case.

From the evidence I have seen the answer is simple: lack of time leading to facile judgements based on rapid reading of material that needed careful analysis. It was our undoing. Contemplating what might have been said further afield about us now that I have seen everything, I am relieved that I'd retired before this happened. And I'm grateful to Ellie, for whom it's been far worse, for obtaining another legal opinion and continuing to trust me.

But resentment gnaws at me.

46

'No! No! Sentence first – verdict afterwards'
– Lewis Carroll

Running through my head is this judgement passed by the senior partner in 2002:

> *My concern is that* nobody *actually thinks that* any *treatment being given in 1990/91/92 actually did* any good at all – *a point made by Dr Forrester.*

We saw in Chapter 38 how it was based on the verdict of Dr Forrester, an expert witness who cited no evidence in his report. He ignored in his 2001 report all the evidence accruing from the 1960s onwards in peer-reviewed specialist and mainstream journals from centres of excellence throughout the world that vascular risk factor management may slow the progress of dementia.

Although we know Carl hadn't had any major strokes before seeing Dr White in October 1993 we don't know whether she found any focal neurological signs of, say, unnoticed minor strokes contributing to his dementia which might have been prevented by earlier treatment of his vascular risk factors. The four pages of her notes where she would have recorded such findings are missing. But something led her to conclude – even before the supporting brain scan results – that Carl had an atherosclerotic (form of vascular) dementia.

The literature up to the present has firmed up the evidence for the contribution of vascular risk factors to the development of dementia and is in the public domain.

Sally Beare's *50 Secrets of the World's Longest Living People*[51] is based on the evidence, known and published by experts before 1990, of longevity and cognitive health in isolated communities following a simple lifestyle and a Mediterranean diet or one of its variants, like the inhabitants of the Italian hill village of Campodimele. Although, predictably, the explanation was partly genetic[52] lifestyle factors were also shown to play a major part.[53] The younger inhabitants of the Japanese island Okinawa who adopted the Western diet of its American occupiers during World War II went on to develop, amongst other things, their patterns of cardiovascular disease and cognitive impairment[54] from which their ancestors had been remarkably free.

And, consistent with these findings, studies based on Scandinavian twin registers identified potentially modifiable dietary as well as genetic factors in the development of dementia including the Alzheimer type.[55,56] Morris (2009) reviewed the epidemiological evidence for the role of nutrition in Alzheimer's disease.[57]

Worth mentioning here are some studies showing some cognitive improvement with the use of lipid lowering agents.[58,59,60] Deschaintre *et al* showed that patients in whom all vascular risk factors were treated declined less rapidly than untreated patients whilst those who had some risk factors treated occupied an intermediate position.[61]

Etminan's meta-analysis (statistical pooling of results) of seven observational studies from different centres provided some support for the value of management of vascular risk factors in lowering the risk of cognitive decline[62]. But the results from large randomised controlled trials of treatment of vascular risk factors in slowing the progress of dementia remained conflicting. So Dr Forrester was right and any expert with a different opinion on this subject of 'intense international research interest'[63] was either wrong or didn't exist (the senior partner's 'Nobody'). Right?

Not exactly. In fact, nowhere near. Various confounding

factors skewing the results of both *negative and positive* findings are advanced by Inzitari et al,[64] by Marler[65] and by Gorelick[66] in Bowler and Hachinsky's *Vascular Cognitive Impairment: Preventable Dementia*.[58]

For example, there is evidence that vascular risk factors need to be targeted much sooner than in established dementia.[55,56,66,67] Studies correlating contemporaneous vascular risk factor levels in subjects with established dementia are capable of yielding misleading results.

An early example of another confounding factor is in Meyer's 1986 study[68]. Treatment of raised blood pressure improved cognition but in some patients lowering the blood pressure too much impaired cognition by reducing the supply of oxygen and nutrients to the brain via the blood.

Richard and Pasquier note in their 2012 review article that the contradictions and inconclusive evidence may be resolved by the findings of Pasquier's large multi-centre COVARAL study on the effect of rigorously controlling all vascular risk factors which are expected soon.[69]

Professor Pasquier's contributions to our understanding of the dementias are matched by the insights she provides on the human consequences of early-onset dementia. She is co-author (the lead author is Francine Ducharme) of a recent article on the difficulties for spouses, including 'the long quest for diagnosis'.[70] In May 2013, in a talk at Imperial College, London (available on YouTube) she spoke, calmly and movingly, of the evidence in France of all the social consequences – including the role reversal of children whose parent develops early-onset dementia.[71] It's not only spouses who end up becoming parents.

By then, faced with the burden of rising dementia rates in ageing populations with high levels of vascular risk factors, UK general recommendations on prevention and management of dementia had become pragmatic: deal with the vascular risk factors a.s.a.p.[72,73,74,75]

I found a clue to how much timely risk vascular risk factor management might have helped Carl in Purandare and Burns's 2005 *Vascular Dementia Factsheet*.[72]

The authors state that the risk factors for vascular dementia are:

> *...potentially controllable by good compliance with prescribed medications (for example tablets to reduce blood pressure) and by improving lifestyle: cessation of smoking, balanced diet and regular exercise.*

They continue:

> *The course of vascular dementia varies considerably. In the early stages, only memory problems and some difficulties with level functioning (for example, problem solving and planning) may be evident. The illness is associated with long periods of stability, interrupted by intermittent worsening.* The progression of the illness depends on the number, severity and control of the underlying vascular risk factors. *Overall, the duration of survival is the same as that for Alzheimer's disease, i.e. around eight years. The cause of death is usually related to the vascular risk factors: for example, stroke or heart attack, often leading to a chest infection.*

So I believe the verdict from an expert such as the one I suggested originally would have been something like this:

> *There was increasing evidence available at the time that vascular risk factor control may slow the progress of vascular dementia, and was necessary to minimise the risk of the strokes – with their own risk of dementia – to which sufferers from both Alzheimer type and vascular*

dementia are prone. Mr Valente's vascular risk factors were potentially controllable at his age by good compliance with lifestyle improvements plus medication if needed. It would be difficult to quantify in any one patient for legal purposes the effect that timely and appropriate management of his vascular risk factors might have had on the disease process itself. However, both the patient and his carer would have benefited from the knowledge that, with occupational stressors removed, they themselves were doing all they could in the light of modern knowledge to keep the disease at bay and enjoy whatever moments of happiness remained for them.

In short, the damage caused by the failure to investigate Carl's condition and manage the vascular risk factors resulted, from a legal standpoint at the time, in 'loss of a chance' of slowing the progress of the dementia, for which a modest amount might have been tagged to an award for pecuniary damages. That is if the solicitors' failure to obtain full evidence of Carl's business finances before it was too late had not robbed them of that chance too.

If you want a job doing, do it yourself. I wish I'd got in touch myself with one or two people I knew for the latest views on the status of the vascular risk factors. And suggested Ellie had a go at obtaining Carl's business records herself for an accountant's view on their significance.

47

*'Blessed is he that expecteth nothing
for he shall not be disappointed'*
– Alexander Pope, 1688–1744

Four years of legal activity and expert reports led to a miscarriage of natural justice – what feels right and fair to the ordinary man:

- For this couple whose success and decency were besmirched and who ended up with nothing, like the majority of clinical negligence complainants.
- For the wife whose sufferings as a 'secondary' victim increased as the dementia took hold, whilst her husband's pain was eased by loss of insight.
- For their conscientious doctor, who was trying hard but, being human, had made the sad mistake of going miles down the wrong diagnostic road in the vain hope that the cure would be around the next corner and then the next, and so on.
- For the wife's cousin who, in trying to support them with her specialist knowledge and some medico-legal experience, saw her academic achievements, research and professionalism debased, and her integrity impugned.

From late dementia diagnosis to the ultimate tragedy, the death of your child, denial of truth and natural justice befall the majority of medical accident victims.

In America the picture is much the same as here despite that nation's proclivity for litigation. It is estimated from systematic research[76,77] that thousands of Americans die every year as a result of the treatment they receive in hospital, many next-of-kin not even realising that a mistake has been made.

When they do suspect it, they demand answers because they don't want it to happen to anyone else. They want comfort from knowing that the hurt they have suffered has helped others. Most of the time it's not about the money. Money can't give you back what's been taken from you, whether it's three lost years, your healthy kidney that's been removed instead of the diseased one, or your child's life.

But money is the currency of justice for the victim. Ellie didn't want money for herself: she wanted to give it to the Alzheimer's Society. Three-quarters of their fifty thousand pounds had ended up in a major bank (a mere drop in the ocean to them). The species of bank manager who would once have stopped the debt in its tracks by summoning Carl into his office and demanding an explanation had become extinct.

You can't put the clock back. Only reflect on how things went wrong – and learn from them.

48

First do no harm

How could a doctor get it wrong for so long? Everybody knows the symptoms of dementia. You might ask why someone so ignorant should be practising.

But Dr Bromwich wasn't ignorant. He was a conscientious doctor who made a mistake as, sadly, we all do.

As a final year medical student he would have been ready to impress the examiners with his knowledge of the differential diagnosis of pre-senile memory loss and the importance of full and early investigation in these cases, maybe working into his answer a couple of rare syndromes with long names. And, as a senior partner, he would have tutored his trainees on the management of memory loss in general practice. Would have told them, I'm sure, that the main things to consider are early-onset dementia and depression, how to make the difficult distinction between them, what primary investigations to do, and when to seek specialist advice.

He made a mistake in this couple's case: he failed to practise what, we can safely assert, he knew from his medical training and preached to his trainees – with nightmare consequences for them. And, as we have seen, he was in denial afterwards because a doctor must never make a mistake. Look at the outcome: the opposite of what anyone who goes into medicine wants to achieve.

As the Harvard study shows,[78,79] doctors, being human, do make mistakes, sometimes with tragic consequences. The large majority go unrecorded as such and only a minuscule number of the others ever obtain redress. This pattern is replicated throughout the world with doctors, patients, their representatives and politicians all struggling to find a solution that is both practicable and fair to all.

My mistake

First do no harm is a fundamental principle underpinning medical education. I can remember in my last term of basic medical science, before we began to see patients, attending an introductory lecture on drugs and prescribing by the Professor of Pharmacology. We were excited, getting closer to the real stuff after eighteen months of cramming anatomy, physiology, and biochemistry into our reluctant brains.

He was an entertaining lecturer, a good raconteur with a stock of anecdotes that had us first smiling then laughing. Towards the end he told us a little about drugs A and B. I can't remember what they were but I'll never forget what he said next: 'Never prescribe these drugs together because, if you do, you'll kill the patient.'

And we all fell about laughing at this latest witticism. After we'd subsided he said: 'When I give a similar warning to a group of final year students, they do not laugh. They write it down to make sure they will never make that mistake.'

I got the message, so I thought. I would never make a mistake. Soon afterwards I did.

The patient came into Casualty (as it was called then) with a minor hand infection. I carried out my student duty of taking a history from her and explained to the doctor in charge (qualified for about two years) what I thought should be done. He saw the patient and agreed she needed a penicillin injection. When I got the injection ready the patient told me she thought she might be allergic to penicillin – she'd once come out in a rash.

I should have stopped there and asked for the doctor's advice.

187

But you have to deal with patients quickly in Casualty. The doctor was busy with an emergency by then, there was a queue of people waiting, and dramatic allergic reactions even to penicillin weren't a common problem in those days. That may have been the reason why the doctor didn't ask her about allergies before he wrote her up for the penicillin. None of that excuses my behaviour: I gave the injection and she came out in a widespread rash with wheezing. An injection of adrenaline quickly solved the problem but the patient, understandably pretty unimpressed, told me to my face what she thought of me.

I was lucky to learn my lesson from being publicly chastened by a very much alive patient. If she'd had a fatal anaphylactic shock after leaving the hospital, it could have been via a complaint or a lawsuit brought by her grieving family.

If I had done the right thing, a possible scenario could have been her becoming fed up with having to wait – and wait – until the doctor was free to examine her again. Before then, she might have left without telling anyone because she had to take the kids to the dentist. The hospital's letter to the GP explaining everything may then have escaped attention at the GP surgery.

The outcome then could have been similar to that caused by a different mistake in the management of an apparently minor hand infection also made in a busy Casualty department.[80] On this occasion, a doctor, about three years qualified, did all the right things apart from testing for spread of infection to the deep tissues of the hand. To this day he does not know how he came to omit the test which he knew should have been done. He didn't see the patient again himself. She was seen at follow-up by three more doctors, one her GP, who perpetuated the first doctor's error until she ended up having a finger amputated.

When the first doctor was informed of the outcome in a letter from the patient's solicitor, he was represented by his medical defence association (no longer the case in the NHS). They informed him, in what he described as a chastening interview, that the indefensible claim would be settled out of court reminding him of the human consequences of losing a finger. It took the lawyers representing the five parties a year to settle the question of apportioning responsibility between the first doctor, the other three doctors and the health authority concerned (for employing inexperienced casualty officers).

A near miss

I'll never forget that Monday evening, the end of my thus far uneventful first day at work after I'd qualified. An elderly, ill-looking man came into Casualty complaining that the stuff he was coughing up had been a bit blood streaked over the last few days. He asked if it would wait until Friday when he was due for a check-up of his lung cancer. It felt as if he was whistling in the dark.

I suspected that the tumour was beginning to erode a major blood vessel. It would rupture, he'd have a torrential bleed and die. There was nothing anyone could do about that. It was a question of when. I told him we'd best keep an eye on him overnight and in the morning liaise with his consultant at the cancer hospital. About an hour later, I met the junior doctor coming out of the ward. He said: 'That chap you admitted has just coughed up a load of blood and died.'

Such paradoxical, but not insensitive, relief: he'd sought his last refuge acting on animal instinct that his death was imminent; I'd provided it for him acting on medical training. I'll always wonder whether, if we and the nearby hospitals all had our extra beds in use (something that's not allowed now), I would have trusted to luck that he would last until the morning and sent him home for the night. He would have become the victim of a medical mishap duly reported in the press: 'Man bleeds to death outside hospital after newly qualified doctor sends him home.' And I believe legally I wouldn't have been negligent because we couldn't have prevented it.

A GP has on average ten minutes per patient. For a telling

account of the skill involved in utilising this short time, read Dr Benjamin Daniels' *Confessions of a GP.*[81]

Working on the medical maxim that 'common things occur commonly', GPs will inevitably be right most of the time. The difficulty lies in spotting the odd one out under the circumstances. I remember being warned as a student about the possibility of someone with appendicitis lurking among the victims in an outbreak of gastro-enteritis. About six months after I'd qualified, a young man came into Casualty with symptoms of gastro-enteritis after a curry night out. Wondering if he could be the one with appendicitis, I called in the surgeon who, on balance, agreed. We were right, somewhat to our surprise.

It's much easier to be right in a hospital when help is only a phone call away than it is if you're a GP called to a patient living out in the wilds who makes it very clear to you how inconvenient it would be to spend the night in hospital.

Blood transfusion pitfalls

When I was on duty one evening early in my career in laboratory medicine I was asked to cross match blood for an operation the next morning. The request form stated that the patient's blood group was O Rhesus negative.

I grouped the sample. It was A positive. I repeated the test using other methods – the blood group obstinately remained A positive.

Most mismatched transfusions which can kill patients are caused by careless clerical, not complex technical, errors. There were two possibilities:

1. The blood had been taken from a different patient who was A positive and mislabelled with our patient's name.
2. The blood had been taken from our patient who was A positive; the information that she was O negative was incorrect.

My phone call to the junior doctor brought the retort that he'd taken the blood from the right patient and labelled the sample himself so there had been no mix-up. And she was *definitely* O negative – because the patient's husband, a *consultant haematologist*, said so. Would I mind admitting to my mistake and get on with the job?

No wonder there was a joke in Path Labs that request forms should have a section: 'Please indicate result required.'

This wasn't funny, though. I still had no idea what our patient's blood group really was. If I cross-matched blood for her using the sample provided, there were three possible outcomes:

1. If she was A positive and the sample had come from her she would receive two units of blood cross-matched against her own blood – the object of the exercise.
2. If she was A positive and the sample came not from her but from another A positive patient, she probably would have come to no harm although the two hour cross-matching procedure (as it was then) would have been pointless.
3. If the sample came not from her but from an A positive patient, and she really was O negative – as her consultant haematologist husband said – it could have killed her.

I knew what I had to do. I refused to issue any blood playing a dead bat to the doctor's wrath at having to postpone the operation. The consultants got together the next morning, delivering their verdict soon after:

> *The patient's husband is very sorry for all the inconvenience he's caused by trying to be helpful. He's the one who is O negative and his wife is A positive. He can't understand how he came to make such a simple mistake.*

Mishaps like the third one were rarities in our lab where the highest standards were maintained by everyone from the top brass down but in some places they were accidents which had been waiting to happen. Add to that the inherent risk in medical procedures even when performed with consummate care and skill and the greater risk when they aren't – anything from a doctor having an off day to indefensible negligence.

What is a medical mishap? What is a medical mistake? What is a negligent medical mistake? Surgeon Patrick Riley's good-read novel, *Serious Misconduct*,[82] shows you why the answer isn't simple.

49

Accidents waiting to happen

Have you got the right leg?

People and teams proceed with familiar tasks according to assumptions. In the operating theatre, staff would proceed on the normally dependable assumption that the series of checks that this was the correct leg/hip/kidney/patient had been done. The terrible result when an incorrect assumption wasn't spotted in time was classified by the World Health Organisation (WHO) and the NHS as 'wrong-site surgery' or a 'Never Event': an accident that should never have happened. The WHO's 'Safe Surgery Checklist' is used now in all British hospitals and such accidents have become uncommon.[83]

Organisational deficiencies

In Rosenthal, Mulcahy and Lloyd-Bostock's 1999 book *Medical Mishaps Pieces of the Puzzle*[84], there are two chapters on human error and accidents by Brennan and Leape,[85] medical doctor and co-author of the Harvard Study,[86,87] and by Charles Vincent and James Reason,[88] professors of psychology, who have written extensively on error and accidents in a range of human activities, including medicine, the principles being common to each.

They distinguish between active failures: errors committed by those at the 'sharp end' of a system and latent failures, 'accidents waiting to happen', in the flawed system itself. They state that 'the distinction between active and latent failures owes a great deal to

Mr Justice Sheen's observations in 1987 regarding the capsizing of a British ship the *Herald of Free Enterprise*' in Zeebrugge harbour after the crew's failure to shut the bow doors:

> *...At first sight the faults which led to this disaster were the...errors of omission on the part of the Master, the Chief Officer and the assistant bosun...But a full investigation into the circumstances of the disaster leads inexorably to the conclusion that the underlying or cardinal faults lay higher up in the Company...From top to bottom the body corporate was infected with the disease of sloppiness.*[89]

An avoidable tragedy

The aviation industry's record on accident prevention has been much better than that of health organisations as an airline pilot would tragically discover.

His wife was being anaesthetised for a minor operation when she developed severe laryngeal spasm, a known complication. The muscles in the larynx (voice box) contract and can block the airway completely. The anaesthetist was unable to intubate (insert a tube into the windpipe to keep the airway open) or get the larynx to relax. It became the 'Can't intubate, can't ventilate' emergency where making an air opening into the windpipe lower down the neck, e.g. by a tracheostomy, risks notwithstanding, was the only way of getting air into the lungs. A team from the adjacent operating theatre came to help and the theatre staff on the periphery of the action had the instrument tray ready.

But the doctors, working desperately on the actions which normally succeeded, seemed unaware of the passage of time. That appears to be why the Difficult Airway Society's guidelines, which would have prevented the death of this previously fit mother of a young family, had not been followed. Her husband could see through his grief that these doctors, nurses and theatre staff weren't bad people. Unlike flight crews, they had not been drilled in leadership, communication, and the automatic application of their theoretical knowledge and skills to a rapidly changing situation.

He channelled that grief into a full professional investigation of what went wrong and how a repeat could be prevented:[90,91] a system of ensuring that those taking action were made fully aware, amongst other things, of the passage of time during a desperate emergency needing fast action. In 2007 he founded an organisation, the Clinical Human Factors Group, which campaigns for the NHS to emulate the airline industry 'so that others may learn and even more may live'.

50

'The appliance of science'
– Advertising slogan for Zanussi washing machines, 1982

Backroom boys

When Ellie asked me to go through Carl's notes in autumn 1998 after she had received the Complaints Manager's response, I had recently finished reports on two cases of pre-senile dementia, both caused by occupational exposure to chemicals which can affect brain biochemistry.

A consultant psychologist's opinion was also vital in both cases. Detailed measurements of all aspects of cognitive function, including memory, reasoning and decision making are the psychology equivalent of Path Lab tests, X-rays, scans, ECGs and all the other back-up measurements doctors ask for. And the appliance of any science, whether it is formal psychology tests or blood tests or the assessment of research findings has its difficulties and pitfalls which need not only thorough understanding of the subject but also skilful communication to overcome.

Never jump to conclusions

Not long before I retired I was asked to provide a report on a Path Lab worker who had contracted hepatitis B, a known occupational hazard in her job usually due to contact with blood from infected patients.

Laboratory procedures had been tightened up after a hepatitis B outbreak in an Edinburgh hospital in 1969 – 1970 in which a number of dialysis patients, two transplant surgeons, and two

Path Lab staff died. Sporadic cases continued to occur. The legal question in this case was whether procedural lapses had, on the balance of probability, caused the hepatitis.

One of the problems had been failure to wear gloves during the preparation of routine samples for analysis because infection can occur through handling samples from unsuspected hepatitis carriers. The report by an expert in liver disease, engaged by the defendant health authority's solicitors, explained that one in eight hundred blood samples would come from an unsuspected hepatitis carrier.

Although his figure was correct, he quite properly didn't go outside his field of expertise into laboratory medicine to give an opinion on its significance. You might assume from these long odds that exposure to the virus was very unlikely. And you would be wrong. A normal throughput in an NHS Path Lab of around two hundred and fifty to three hundred samples per day (readily quantifiable from laboratory records) equates to handling one unsuspected hepatitis sample every three days or so. As I explained in my report for the claimant's solicitors that constitutes regular, not low, exposure to the hepatitis B virus.

Levels of probability

I was once asked to give a report for a Trade Union's solicitors in a case where one of their members believed that exposure to an industrial toxin at work had caused her cancer. She had developed it at a much younger than expected age (suggestive of an additional environmental effect such as the one in question) and two small epidemiological studies in peer-reviewed journals seemed to support it. It was the sort of case where the patient's intuition might be proved right a decade later, but nobody could say for certain right now.

I concluded that, *on the balance of probability*, there was no connection between their client's occupational exposure to the chemical and her cancer, guessing that she would feel aggrieved by not being taken seriously. The union agreed to fund a report from an epidemiologist to assess the strength of the evidence from the two studies. As it turned out, he came to the same conclusion as I had.

Not the outcome she'd hoped for but she and her union had been given a dispassionate expert assessment which might prove helpful for future research and for others. In that sense alone she had received far more than many claimants.

Use and misuse of statistics

A couple lost their first two babies in 1996 and 1998 to sudden infant death syndrome, a.k.a. SIDS and 'cot death'. The mother stood trial in 1999, was found guilty on a majority verdict of smothering both babies and imprisoned. The victim became the wrongdoer. Their third baby was placed in foster care.[92]

Crucial laboratory evidence of an infection in the second baby was not available to either prosecution or defence until the second appeal in January 2003. And at the trial, a professor of paediatrics had made a startling claim. He put the chance of two cot deaths happening in one family at one in seventy-three million, occurring only once in a hundred years. The extent to which this influenced the jury will never be known.

He had gone outside his field of specialist expertise into epidemiology to make his facile assertion. It was shown to be fallacious by Dr Stephen Watkins[93] whose speciality of epidemiology requires a level of mathematical ability not necessarily found in other branches of medicine. His stance was backed by a press release from the Royal Statistical Society.[94]

Assuming for the sake of argument that SIDS is a random event, two will occur in the same family somewhere in England once every *seven* years. But they aren't necessarily random events: the syndrome's (partly understood) causes and risk factors such as poor living conditions and smokers in the household can increase the likelihood. Articles on the topic in peer-reviewed mainstream paediatric, as well as epidemiological, journals are testimony to the actual frequency of recurrent cot deaths in a single family. According to Dr Watkins,[93] two cot deaths would be expected to occur in the same family somewhere in England on average once every *year-and-a-half.*

In addition, the professor's calculation was conducive to what The Royal Statistical Society described as 'a serious error of logic known as the Prosecutor's Fallacy'.[94] They explained:

> *The jury needs to weigh up two competing explanations for the babies' deaths: SIDS or murder. Two deaths by SIDS or two murders are each quite unlikely, but one has apparently happened in this case. What matters is the relative likelihood of the deaths under each explanation, not just how unlikely they are under one explanation (in this case SIDS, according to the evidence as presented).*

The appeal judges ruled that the conviction was unsafe and the mother was released after three years in prison. She'd made good friends not only among staff but also among inmates whose raw humanity and sense of fairness were as supportive to her as her professionalism was to them.

The appliance of science came too late to prevent an outcome as tragic as the events that provoked it. Her living third child would call to Daddy or Nanny for comfort until the day came when she heard him call out for her, his mother. But her mind and body, exhausted by catastrophic events not of her making, could function no longer. One night in 2007 she fell asleep never to wake again, leaving behind her father, her husband and the child who'd begun to call her Mummy.

51

Without prejudice

What makes an expert witness?

The majority of cases which come to lawyers are to some extent arguable. It isn't difficult for lawyers to conclude from an expert report that, on the balance of probability, the doctor didn't made a negligent mistake. Someone once commented to me that a doctor who could write ambiguous or, as occasionally happens, tendentious reports couldn't be trusted. To my surprise quick as a flash I found myself replying: 'They wouldn't treat their patients like that.'

I'd hit on the problem.

Medical expert witnesses are reporting on a doctor who has made a mistake with disastrous consequences, perhaps one they could imagine themselves making under those circumstances. Such mistakes shouldn't be allowed to jeopardise a good doctor's career. You can't put the clock back.

What makes a good expert witness?

We saw earlier that the specialist expert who got to the heart of Carl's problem was the psychologist I'd recommended. He was considered unsatisfactory by our lawyers because he had 'no medico-legal experience' i.e. he'd never had to appear in court to defend his opinions. I suspect they pictured a hectoring barrister making mincemeat of him. Or a despairing barrister giving up after this type of exchange:

Counsel: *'Was the door open or was it shut?'*
Expert: *'That's a very interesting question. Actually, the door was slightly ajar, to an extent that was determined by a most unusual set of circumstances. Let's imagine for a moment that...'*
Counsel: *'No further questions.'*

Providing expert evidence

Biological events aren't open or shut, to the despair of learned Counsel in the famous 1960s Lydney murder trial. The case hinged on the date of death according to the common bluebottle's egg-laying habits versus witnesses' recollections. The defence had engaged a professor of entomology to pick holes in the prosecution evidence concerning the date on which the bluebottle maggots would have hatched.

As the late Professor Keith Simpson explains in his memoirs,[95] things didn't turn out that way. The defence entomologist, a professorial figure with wispy hair and a ready smile, began by agreeing with the prosecution expert on when the maggots would have hatched. The defence Counsel's subsequent endeavours to elicit something from him favourable to the defence merely allowed him to expound on his beloved subject:

> *'Maggots are curious little devils. Suppose this is a dead body,'* he said, placing a matchbox on the edge of the witness box, *'and you have a hundred maggots.'* He threw out his hands expansively. *'Ninety-nine will make their way towards the body, but the hundredth little devil, he'll turn the other way.'*

Smiles all round, apart from the judge whose lips twitched slightly, and the frowning defending Counsel who said: 'No further questions.'

The case is described in another forensic pathologist's

memoirs.[96] Yes, the defence and prosecution experts were agreed on the crucial question of the normal hatching rate of bluebottle maggots – but the question lost sight of in the theatre of the criminal court was whether it could have been affected by the unusually hot weather at the time. (Fortunately for the defendant capital punishment had ended not long before.)

It's the sort of question that's normally resolved in academic discussions between experts. Or between solicitors and expert witnesses before the case gets to court. That's how truth comes to light.

The iconic expert

If a debatable question comes up in open court it can lead to 'experts never agreeing' – and the verdict going to the one with the biggest reputation who clearly, concisely and convincingly states his – not necessarily correct – opinion.

The supreme example, cited by some even now, of such an expert is the iconic Sir Bernard Spilsbury, the subject of barrister Andrew Rose's biography *Lethal Witness*.[97] Spilsbury's evidence sent to the gallows more than one person who should have been declared not guilty. The final letter from one prisoner in the condemned cell ends: 'Never mind, dad, don't worry. I am a martyr to Spilsburyism.' Another, acquitted on Sir Bernard's idiosyncratic but unsuccessfully challenged opinion, went on to kill two more people, three if you include the murderer himself. A contemporary forensic pathologist, Professor Sir Sydney Smith, wrote in his memoirs:[98]

> *One might almost hope that there will never be another Bernard Spilsbury.*

Lord Woolf tried to tackle, amongst other things, the dilemma of disagreement between experts in his 1999 reforms.[99,100] Dr Miller, the only one of the specialist expert witnesses to have done so, had attended a course on them to make sure that his reports were in accordance with current legal requirements.

Lord Woolf made a number of recommendations. One was a meeting of experts on both sides to clarify what they were agreed on. Shortly after this, I wrote a report on a man exposed to toxic chemicals at work. One of his complaints was dermatitis, in which it can be difficult to apportion responsibility between occupational and non-occupational causes. The defence and prosecution dermatologists put their heads together and produced this:

We are AGREED that this man has dermatitis.

Another recommendation was for a single joint expert acceptable to both sides. It's not hard to envisage such an arrangement leading to a miscarriage of justice. If expert witnesses always maintained the highest standards of dispassionate expert analysis there wouldn't be a problem. But, as Dr Stephen Watkins observes in his book, *The Politics of a Profession,*[101] doctors are human and, whilst drawing the line at blatant corruption, do not constantly maintain the heights of iron integrity.

A disincentive to an expert witness maintaining 'iron integrity' was, until recently, expert witness immunity. All witnesses, according to common law going back to the seventeenth century used to be given protection against reprisals for telling the truth. Or lies – unless the then powers that be thought they'd rule that out by making witnesses swear, on pain of going to Hell, to tell the truth, the whole truth and nothing but the truth. Or facile judgements on complex evidence.

Expert witness immunity ended in 2011 on a three to two majority verdict of the law lords.[102] To my knowledge, one expert witness has been taken to court – after being persuaded by the expert for other side into changing the evidence she gave in court from that in her report.

52

The scales of justice

Clinical negligence is a difficult speciality with scant rewards and the occasional spectacular success, nicely put by Charles Lewis in the Introduction to *Clinical Negligence:*[103]

> *Many of the solicitors who are qualified to do the work form a tight-knit group, striving to outdo their rivals with some striking victory, and ever on the look-out for new ways of extending the boundaries of the medical negligence claim.*

Attempts to strike a balance between what is fair to the victim, to the doctor and to the community feel like trying to square the circle. Read *Medical Mishaps Pieces of the Puzzle* (it's not all heavy going) for glimmers of hope:[104]

Alternative Dispute Resolution

Fifty-odd years ago we were taught that that there was a condition called 'compensation neurosis': the patient's symptoms would not disappear until her claim was settled. I cannot recall any reference being made to the merit of such claims. Complaints procedures were rudimentary then and litigation was an option only for the rich.

The number of patients seeking redress after medical mishaps increased after the inception of the NHS. Doctors had to be members of one of the medical protection societies who would conduct their defence in the event of litigation.

Each year a representative sample of cases was published anonymously in the society's annual report. The cases fell into three groups: without foundation (either try-ons or disappointed expectations), arguable, and indefensible. Doctors were able to learn from these cases until the NHS reforms of 1990 when medical negligence claims became the responsibility of the health authorities. An unfortunate side effect was that most NHS doctors' supply of these instructive case histories ended.

As diagnosis and treatment became more effective, patients' expectations rose. But no procedure is completely risk free. Being the unlucky one is, *from a statistical standpoint,* exactly like winning a raffle: it's unlikely to be you but it will be someone. When the unlucky one asks: 'Why me?' an explanation lets them get on with their lives. It's perfectly possible: I've done it for a number of people.

Someone once asked me to do a report for a clinical negligence lawyer, both of us working pro bono. The patient, after treatment of her overactive thyroid by a consultant physician, had suffered the well-known but uncommon and serious complication of pressure build-up in the eye sockets. It runs its course, only rarely needing a major operation, orbital decompression, in which the tissues around the eyeball are removed to relieve the pressure and save the patient's sight.

The patient was caring for her terminally ill husband at the time. Her GP had referred her promptly to the ophthalmologist who'd rightly advised a wait-and-see policy but in a very offhand way: 'It'll get better. Off you go. Keep on taking the tablets.' She was the unlucky one in whom it didn't get better.

Her GP was deaf to her complaints of increasing pain because the specialist had told him that nothing more need be done. But the specialist's implicit assumption when writing to another doctor would have been that if the patient developed very severe pain he would see her again.

In desperation she went into A&E one evening, had emergency eye surgery (orbital decompression) and was told that if she'd left it another week she'd have lost her sight. She was inclined to blame the first doctor: she was a lot sicker after she'd seen him than she was before. And now look what had happened.

By the time I saw her she'd been fobbed off by three health authorities (one for each doctor) instead of being given an explanation. At first I wondered if she could be right to blame the first doctor: occasionally clinicians' interpretation of the Path Lab's thyroid function tests left something to be desired. Perhaps her thyroid hadn't been overactive.

The medical notes told a different story. The right tests had been done, the right conclusions drawn and one of two reasonable treatment options given. She was simply the unlucky one who'd developed the thyroid eye disease.

The ophthalmologist's reply to the GP should, instead of the terse note confirming the thyroid eye disease, have expressed some regard for the unfortunate patient's circumstances, emphasise his willingness to see her again if her symptoms worsened and explain that to the patient as well. And the GP, when the patient complained to him of increasing pain, should have contacted the ophthalmologist for advice.

The patient didn't have a case against them because her sight was saved, more by her own common sense than good management by the doctors. When the truth had sunk in, the patient said: 'Why couldn't somebody have explained it like that?'

Irrespective of whether they were the victims of bad luck or bad management, people want to know the truth: they don't want what they went through to happen to anyone else.

But complainants are less likely to be told the truth than to be stone-walled by a health authority whose default position is: 'Never admit liability'.

Imagine this scenario: all children have experienced the guilt and shame of spoiling something their parent held dear. They run the gamut, starting with the defence, true or false, that it wasn't their fault:

1. What were you doing? *Nothing.*
2. Tell the truth and shame the devil. *I picked up your glass vase to help you…*
3. Say you're sorry. *Says sorry to call halt to proceedings.*
4. Show me you're sorry. *Offers to dig buttercups out of the lawn/wash up/clean car/vacuum carpets/forego pocket money.*
5. Let's forget it. *Tears and hugs.* Humanity.

We can equate the child's responses in the first paragraph to the post-complaint defensive replies from health authorities:

1. *Nothing* = 'Don't admit liability.'
2. *I moved your glass vase to help you* = 'The doctors did everything they could.'
3. *Says sorry to call halt to proceedings* = 'We are sorry that you feel…'
4. *Offers to make amends* = 'Lessons have been learned.'

Although this last could be a contrite rather than a default response it still begs the question of why things hadn't been changed sooner. And there isn't a fifth stage. The mistake, negligent or not, of an individual in a system conducive to it doesn't necessarily stimulate management improvement: 'It was medical/nursing/driver/pilot/staff error.' End of.

Whilst the term 'compensation neurosis' might have become obsolete, money still remains the law's currency of redress. Some countries have 'no fault compensation schemes' but even these expensive arrangements have their injustices. All claims, irrespective of outcome, are a burden on the taxpayer, and policy – what the country can afford – inevitably comes into the equation.

But concern grew in legal and medical circles about the number and nature of medical mishaps, and the lack, not only of redress for the victim, but also of protocol reviews by the health authorities. A good example is that of the doctor whose mistake caused the loss of a patient's finger. He never met her, as he would have liked, to explain and apologise. He felt it would have been a good thing because it could have allowed her to work through her anger, and him to work through his guilt. The doctors concerned never got together to work out how between them they had made such an appalling error. Her compensation probably wasn't commensurate with the enormity of the injury caused by the mistake.[105]

Linda Mulcahy, Professor of Law at London School of Economics, addressed the question of what complainants actually wanted. The commonest responses were: 'I wanted the truth', 'I wanted them to say sorry' and – one that I think we've all heard – 'I didn't want this to happen to anyone else'.

Her 1995 pilot scheme on behalf of the Department of Health paved the way for mediation after medical mishaps. It 'facilitates settlements involving more than financial compensation: explanations, review of protocols and a promise of full discussion at board level',[106] and was followed in 1996 by the NHS Complaints Procedure.[107]

A woman in the pilot scheme received something more precious than money, all she'd ever wanted and waited for, the knowledge of where her stillborn baby was buried.[108] It was a couple of years after the Good Samaritan, Ellie, had given a stranger, Freda, that same knowledge while the charity SANDS (Stillbirth and Neonatal Death Society) ensured that what Ellie did for Freda was made law, binding professionals to do likewise.

Something more precious than money was at last being weighed on the scales of justice.

53

*'There is but one law for all,
the law of humanity, justice, equity – the law of nature'*
– Edmund Burke, 1729–1797
The Impeachment of Warren Hastings

A few years after Carl's case ended, I was acting as an informal advocate to a woman who'd been denied a widow's pension. Her husband had received a disability pension because the tuberculosis contracted at work had left him with severe lung damage. The question when awarding the widow's pension was whether the lung damage, including the lung cancer (listed on his death certificate) had been caused by the tuberculosis. The pension's expert said it hadn't and I rated the connection as arguable at best. But, upset by the letter's impersonal, peremptory tone, the widow saw the refusal as unfair.

I sensed that she would have seen my scientific caution as betrayal if I'd told her my rating of her chances then. I simply explained that it would take some time to get the case heard and asked her if she felt up to it. She was. When I researched her late husband's medical records and peer-reviewed journals, there was more evidence than I'd expected that the tuberculosis could have been a contributory factor to his lung cancer.

The widow appealed against the decision on that basis. But it was only my opinion in a speciality other than mine. It would be up to the tribunal, chaired by a lawyer, to decide. By the time of the hearing a year later the widow's position was that she didn't mind about the outcome: being listened to was what mattered, not the money.

The chairman explained that the (inquisitorial) proceedings were less formal than in the courts – so we hadn't needed to turn up in our best clothes. They took evidence from the widow and the charity's pension expert, then moved on to the spokesman for the pensions people. He said the lung cancer was caused not by his work but by smoking forty cigarettes a day...He got no further. The widow turned abruptly, not to the tribunal, but to him: 'That's not true! He never did!'

She was allowed to have her say. She described her late husband's modest smoking habit of one per day after his main meal; how he'd buy a packet of ten cigarettes a week handing the remaining three out to his friends in the pub every Friday; how he'd stopped smoking completely some years before he died. Exactly as she'd told me.

I rifled through the files knowing the evidence in there of his actual smoking habits was exactly as his widow described. When we came out to wait for the tribunal's findings, she said: 'I've blown it and I don't care. It wasn't true what he said.'

She hadn't blown it. The tribunal found in her favour. The chairman's written findings referred to the evidence, *especially that of the appellant*, which had convinced the tribunal.

The tribunal had listened and judged the evidence according to the law of humanity, justice and equity. It's a law that can become obscured in the adversarial system of the courts, both criminal and civil.

54

Useful advice

Imagine this. A mother of a young child is busy downstairs when it occurs to her that it's too quiet upstairs.

She calls out: 'Johnnie, what are you doing up there?'

'Nothing!'

She has the dinner to cook and a lot on her mind so she yells: 'Well, stop it then!'

Johnnie, who's good with his hands, is making a birthday present for his mother, a box divided into sections to hold her sewing cottons. It looked easy to him. But he's cut the cardboard in not quite the right places so the inside sections won't slot into each other. He's using the wrong type of glue for the outer parts which won't stick together – as his father could have told him. He's sitting behind the bedroom door: originally to stop his mother barging in and spoiling her surprise but now it's because he's spilt glue on the carpet. The outcome depends on how and when his mother, driven by suspicion, demands, forces or negotiates an entry.

The mother in this encounter isn't a passive recipient: she holds the key to achieving the best outcome. It's the same for a patient or their carer. Your doctor might be capable and well-meaning but, being human like Johnnie, he's neither infallible nor possessed of consistent iron integrity. A year after the specialist had made the formal dementia diagnosis, Carl's GP wrote an open letter that he knew was intended for organisations like the local ratings department still labelling Carl's first dementia symptoms as anxiety-depression caused by his business problems.

Add to medical errors the inherent complication rate in any medical procedure or normal physiological event. Childbirth is an example of how things can go suddenly, unpredictably, and tragically wrong with the best will in the world.

Once a mistake is made, normal human thought processes are apt to perpetuate it. It may be the same doctor or even a series of doctors seeing the patient on different occasions. Unless someone takes a fresh look at it as did a different doctor on seeing Carl for the first time.

Ellie assumed that the GP would see Carl after she'd been to the GP herself about him – as was his stated intention. Nothing happened, as we know, yet this was the vital time for action.

What else could she have done?

Useful tips

Never take anything for granted. Once you're out of the room the doctor's mind is on the next patient, a call that's just come in, or any number of things like not feeling well himself. He may not return to your problem, however good his intentions, without a reminder. Think of the times when you've forgotten to make a note of something important because you were distracted. Don't let time drift by.

If you don't feel satisfied, talk to family, friends and neighbours – find a link to someone in one of the health care professions. They'll advise you or know someone who can. The few clinical negligence complainants who do achieve a fair resolution have often been pointed in the right direction by a professional.

Try to define your exact concern. You might have thought: I want to know what's wrong, of course. I've been on/got my friend to go on the internet. Is it dementia, depression, brain tumour, hypothyroidism or Marchiafava-Bignami syndrome? Tell me, you're the doctor. And the doctor will fixate on what feels to him like your implicit message: You don't know, do you, doctor? I'm having to tell you everything.

So you may get short shrift, especially if you go in armed with a sheaf of computer print-outs that you brandish in his face.

Be as specific as you can. Ellie's real concern was: 'We need to know if Carl's likely to get better soon because of the legislation affecting the business.' Before you see the doctor, memorise your questions and write them down on a piece of paper that preferably stays in your pocket.

If you are the one with the problem, ask the doctor if you can bring someone in with you, preferably a health professional with some understanding of what's being said. Their brief is not to catch the doctor out but to listen in case you miss or misinterpret something. If the problem is your partner's symptoms and he's agreeable, ask to see the doctor together. Two heads are better than one. Or, if all parties are approaching the matter in a spirit of honest inquiry, three heads are better than two.

Seeing a different doctor in the same practice can be helpful: either by engineering it somehow or asking for a second opinion. Or, if you can afford it, a private opinion from an appropriate specialist. You aren't paying to jump the NHS queue: you are paying for an hour of a specialist's time, not ten minutes with a harassed GP. And you shouldn't have to wait long to be seen.

If you can't afford it, then you would be thinking of the most appropriate organisation or charity such as the Patients' Association and specific medical charities which provide quality information, guidance and support. For example, Carl's illness was causing both marital and business problems. The charity for problems between couples, Relate, has psychiatrists they can call on: for instance, where the conflict could be caused by illness. They are prepared to see one partner alone if the other is uncooperative.

What's right for you
These tips are also useful if you have been given a diagnosis but are stuck at the stage of deciding which treatment option suits you best. You need to fully understand the risks and benefits of each

as they apply to you. It can take time especially when you aren't in the best state of mind for rational decision making. But it's a decision that the doctor can't make for you if it comes down to one of personal preference – which it often does.

Going back to Carl's case, for example, depending on the findings he should either have been given a diagnosis or been told he had a memory problem that they would have to keep an eye on. They would have made their own decision about closing the business but Ellie would have phoned me about Carl having to see the specialist.

Knowing about his father dying young of a heart attack and his mother having the first of her several strokes at young age, I would have asked about cholesterol, blood pressure, family history of diabetes, etc and wondered about vascular cognitive impairment. I'd have discovered their liking for Mediterranean food, explained about diet and cholesterol, and suggested a specialist who could have advised on all the vascular risk factors.

One size doesn't fit all

It isn't a simple question of defining for, say, cholesterol or blood pressure a rigid cut-off point based on population studies above which any individual whose level on one occasion exceeds it should receive a particular medication. That approach reminds me of a passage in Monica Dickens's book *One Pair of Feet*[109] about a newspaper astrology column foretelling an event at mid-week which would alter her life:

> *...I could only hope that the prophecy was also fulfilled for the million other children of the sign of Taurus. It was a beautiful thought to think of all our fortunes turning simultaneously, like furrows in a ploughed field, and leading on up to better things until at the weekend...*

It's not a flippant comparison. Professor Durrington in *Hyperlipidaemia: Diagnosis and Treatment* writes:

Diagnosis…is not simply a matter of disease classification …there can be no single level of cholesterol which for all individuals necessitates a particular course of action. [110]

Day-to-day variation in the individual, [110] the precision of the laboratory tests [110,111] and the presence of other vascular risk factors may alter the significance of a single measurement of any risk factor sufficiently to affect a recommendation on medication. Statins save lives but like any drug they can have side effects so they aren't for everyone. A trial of simple measures should come first [112,113] followed by a repeat test.

I have a friend, a retired medical laboratory analyst, who's measured cholesterol levels in thousands of blood samples knowing the reasons for the tests. His own cholesterol level used to be too high and he loves Mediterranean cuisine and sea food (good) and fine cheeses (bad). He couldn't bear to give up the cheese so he takes a low dose of a statin which counteracts the effect of the saturated fat in the cheese. He has no side effects from the statin and he's happy.

So can you eat as much butter, cream, full fat cheese, sausages, pork pies, etc as you like and just increase the dose of the statin? No, because either the drug won't manage to compensate or you'll suffer from a side effect of either the drug or the diet. Some people adopt the treat-yourself-once-a-week approach to avoid constantly bombarding their liver with harmful instructions to make more cholesterol. The same principle applies to any risk factor.

What matters is being able to choose the compromise that suits you best based on common sense and good information.

Securing your rights

It's comforting to know how many legal professionals are prepared to give advice, or even take on their case pro bono, when someone feels they haven't had redress after a mishap.

This is where I failed Carl and Ellie. Instead of finding a firm of solicitors, we should have asked around for a lawyer, preferably with some clinical negligence expertise, who could have advised us informally. The other option was the Patient's Association or another similar charity.

Ellie might have been helped to draft another letter to the Complaints Manager, drawing attention, for example, to the failure to inform her of her options, despite it being out of time, for pursuing the matter further. There were public interest issues for any health authority in such a case:

- Was this an isolated error or part of the doctor's general unfitness to practise?
- Is the index of suspicion of dementia too low generally among the health authority's doctors?
- Is there undue delay generally in doing the formal psychological tests for determining fitness to drive?

We'll never know how strong the financial side would have looked had all the information on Carl's business finances been obtained. Get as much information as you can for yourself. When, some years ago, obstetric patients were put in charge of their own notes they generally looked after them better than the hospital did. Ellie got the relevant parts of Carl's GP notes from the practice herself. It cost fifty pounds and took a week – nothing like the solicitors' rigmarole. With Power of Attorney, she could have obtained Carl's business records herself.

Difficulties can arise even with help
Shortly before Carl's case, I did a pro bono report on a man with dementia caused by occupational exposure to toxic chemicals. He had been repeatedly refused a disability pension. At first the organisation's voluntary worker refused to submit it to the Commissioner on the grounds that a famous teaching hospital

professor's opinion, the opposite of mine, had to be right. Undeterred by her lack of either medical or legal qualifications to judge expert medical evidence, she had based her verdict on rank.

With forceful persuasion from the man's wife she relented. The Commissioner referred it, in no uncertain terms, to a (last chance) Medical Appeals Tribunal. They told us as soon as we entered the room, led by a young barrister acting pro bono, that we were banging on open doors and found in the man's favour.

When all that matters is candour, guile takes over as this ultimate of tragedies shows.

Three weeks after Ellie saw Dr Bromwich about Carl, a ten-year-old boy died from the rare but readily treatable Addison's disease. A consultant paediatrician had suspected it the previous autumn, after the boy had been hospitalised for what was thought to be severe gastro-enteritis. He recommended a blood test that would have confirmed it, one done regularly in general hospital Path Labs like the one I used to work in, and that if the boy had another attack of sickness he should be admitted to hospital.

The test wasn't done, seemingly because of communication failure between the hospital and the GPs. The boy had another attack, becoming so weak that he had to be carried to the bathroom. The GP agreed, on her second visit to him in one day, to admit him to hospital allegedly after a heated discussion with his frantic parents. She said an ambulance wasn't the best means of transport for him. The distraught father drove his critically ill child the twenty minute journey to the hospital where he died soon afterwards despite desperate attempts in A&E to save him.

The father's attempts to discover the truth were relentlessly thwarted. He was publicly labelled a liar. The victim became the wrongdoer.

In June 1996 the High Court ruled that the doctors did not owe the parents a duty of care, in civil law, to tell the truth about the circumstances of their child's death or to refrain from falsifying his medical records and the case was struck out. This ruling was upheld by the Court of Appeal, by the House of Lords and, in May 2000, by the European Court of Human Rights:[114]

> *Whilst it is* arguable *that doctors had a duty not to falsify medical records under the common law…there was no binding decision of the courts as to the existence of such a duty. As the law stands now, however, doctors have no duty to give parents of a child who died as a result of their negligence a truthful account of the circumstances of the death, nor even to refrain from deliberately falsifying records.*

So in law these parents of a child who died of a diagnosable and treatable illness are without rights. They are complete nonentities in a worse position than Ellie, who was in the bottom league of 'secondary victims'.

A psychiatrist's report on behalf of the boy's parents who were left suffering from what might have been labelled fifty years ago as 'compensation neurosis' states:

> *Should the outcome* [of the civil litigation] *suggest that justice has been done, at least in his* [the father's] *eyes, then his symptoms will gradually recede and he may make a good recovery and return to normal functioning.*

The report quotes the father:

> *I'd like to prove that my wife and I were good parents who took our son to people* who we trusted. *I have a terrible feeling of emptiness…They haven't let me grieve. I won't grieve until this is sorted out.*

It refers to the mother:

My view, therefore, is that this lady does suffer from chronic panic disorder…the fact that her mother suffered from a similar disorder suggests the possibility of a constitutional predisposition…There is little doubt however that the predominant precipitant was the events that followed *her child's death.*

The Radio 4 programme, *Doctor – Tell Me the Truth,* aired on 27th February and 4th March 2012, was fronted by Dr James Reason, Emeritus Professor of Psychology at Manchester University. The mistake itself was not what hurt most.

At the end of the programme the boy's father, ruined financially but with his dignity and integrity unimpeached, said this: 'It's the honesty part they seem not to understand. It's the most fundamental thing.'

55

'The tender leaves of hope'
— William Shakespeare, *King Henry VIII*

The pressure continues for a statutory duty of candour to those who have suffered harm from medical errors as do the campaigns by Martin Bromiley's Clinical Human Factors Group for improvements in the working systems that give rise to them.

For nearly a century since Alois Alzheimer described the first case of the disease that would bear his name the dementias were seen as another infamous neuro-degenerative condition, like Parkinson's disease and multiple sclerosis. The neurologist, a species of physician with an academic turn of mind, would solve the diagnostic puzzle like *The Times* crossword. His solution became the patient's, carer's and GP's problem: coping with a progressively dissolute brain.

The two commonest dementias, vascular and Alzheimer's type, still lie unnecessarily close to the incurable end of the dementia spectrum. The role of vascular and other risk factors in cognitive impairment, even in those with an inherited tendency to it, is well established now in authoritative public information areas – to prevent and, hopefully, to slow the progress of cognitive impairment. And now there is, amongst other things, a blood test for the set of ten phospholipids (fatty substances coming from brain cells) to help estimate your level of risk more accurately and enable you to put in place measures to counteract the damage well before the disease gets going.[115]

And all dementias can be managed to help the patient make

the best of the hand that life has dealt him – just as other chronic conditions like diabetes and rheumatoid arthritis are managed (O'Connor D.W. et al, 1993).[116] Medication that preserves brain cell function in the early stages of dementia for as long as possible is readily available.

That is what medical science has to offer. And in the later stages of dementia simple humanity is restoring meaning and purpose to the lives of those most oppressed by the dead weight of modern society's escalating cognitive demands. Join in a sing-song, share your memories, cuddle a baby, stroke a cat, pat a dog, feed the birds, water the plants, smell the roses and enjoy the warm sun in its heaven. Like the people of Campodimele, which means 'Field of Honey'.

Epilogue

Easter 2014

Dear Carl
I'm thinking of you and Pete enjoying the gingerbread when you and Ellie came to see us about nailing the bastards.

All the way through writing this book, I've kept thinking of the time – it was in the late eighties – when you dropped in on us. We were teasing each other about us measuring cholesterols in our lab and people being told to cut down on animal fat. I said: 'Carl, joking apart, have our activities affected your business?' And you said: 'No, I've had to make changes but it's working out okay.' Only two or three years later the silent strokes in your thinking brain would put paid to your ability to adapt to change.

Carl, we didn't succeed in shoving under the noses of those who said you'd embarked on a disastrous business venture the evidence that your business had been rock solid. You'd always been good with people and good at figures. And they didn't believe anyone thought that treatment of vascular dementia would have done any good at all although I told them that the evidence was there even then that it might have helped you. Now I hear all the time of someone who's got vascular dementia. There was even someone aged ninety-two on television a year ago who was on a cholesterol lowering drug for it. You were fifty-three and you got nothing. I began to pick up bad vibes from the solicitors early on and felt like going in and confronting them but I sensed it might have made them refuse to continue acting for you. We had to see it through to the end.

After you died and the case was lost, Ellie went to a new solicitor to keep her promise to you. I picked up her burden and wrote this book so other people won't have to go through what you two went through – whether it's late diagnosis of dementia or cancer, or an accident that shouldn't have happened, or the absolute worst, the death of your child.

It's Easter now and we've just been watching a programme on the daffodils full of Galanthamine that they're growing on a Welsh hillside to help people like you. This coming autumn we're going to plant wild daffodils on your grave. They will flower next spring and be full of the Galanthamine that helped you so much until they took it and your hopes from you. Now, like the other treatments for dementia, it's available for anyone who needs it.

We've nailed the bastards.

Postscript

'Ich Hab Mich Verloren'
I have lost myself

– Auguste D, 1901

In 1901, almost ninety years before fifty-three-year-old Carl first went to his GP complaining that he was losing his memory and concentration, Dr Alois Alzheimer saw fifty-one-year-old Auguste D because her husband was complaining that she was suffering from something similar. She was losing her memory, was unable to manage her usual household tasks, and had uncharacteristic paranoid outbursts. He could cope no longer.

Since time immemorial it had been recognised that age made you not only physically but also mentally less agile. By the turn of the nineteenth century, however, microscopy, biochemistry and tissue staining methods had advanced enough for doctors to link impaired brain function to atherosclerosis (furring up) of the arteries supplying blood to the brain.

Alzheimer had published his microscopic findings on atherosclerotic (furring up of the arteries, i.e. a type of vascular) dementia in 1899.[117] It would remain for over half a century in the shadow of the relentlessly progressive form of dementia that still bears his name following the presentation at a conference in Germany of his first case seven years later.[118]

Alzheimer didn't name it after himself. Kraepelin, his head of department in Frankfurt, seems to have done that for – and without reference to – him. Kraepelin's reasons were possibly to get his department's ideas on the map as prominently as Pick's in Munich and those of Sigmund Freud and other psycho-analysts.

Not necessarily a bad thing: healthy scepticism and competition between research centres puts the brakes on the excesses to which creative minds can be prone.

Alzheimer himself comes over as a caring clinician, an obsessive searcher for the truth lurking down his microscope, and a family man with a fondness for cigars.[119] His appointment as a psychiatrist and neuropathologist, common in those days, straddled two specialities: something that doesn't happen now because of the overwhelming volume of accumulated information in both. To bridge that gap we are dependent nowadays on another human factor: communication. We saw the consequences of the lack of this essential skill earlier in this book. You don't need much imagination to realise that the aptitudes required for each specialism don't necessarily co-exist in one person.

It was said of Alzheimer by Robert Gaupp, head of the Department of Psychiatry:

> *Alzheimer was a man with a clear head and unusual creative powers who took great pains over his work and had a strong sense for scientific truth.*[120]

But were an inordinate fondness for cigars and spending the evening peering down a microscope all that was significant about Dr, later Professor, Alois Alzheimer? He'd been widowed earlier that year and was now reliant on his sister to bring up their young family.

Whereas Cecilie Alzheimer had died after a long illness that destroyed her body but left her mind and spirit intact, Auguste D's illness had destroyed her mind and spirit, then progressed to the primitive part of her brain that controls basic bodily functions.

So it's easy to imagine empathy between the two widowers. Alzheimer's meticulous notes on Auguste D reveal both his clinical skills and his compassion. And, although her unkempt body (no longer controlled by her brain) and paranoid rage wouldn't endear her to many, their human interaction when he examines her is revealing of them both:

> Alzheimer: *On what street do you live?*
> Auguste D: *I can tell you, I must wait a bit.*
> Alzheimer: *What did I ask you?*
> Auguste D: *Well, this is Frankfurt am Main* [correct but not what he asked her]
> Alzheimer: *On what street do you live?*
> Auguste D: *Waldemarstrasse, not, no...* [not quite right: it's her daughter's address and she's anxious.]

Next he shows her a key, a pencil, and a book that she names correctly. But when he asks her to name them again she's forgotten:

> Auguste D: *I don't know, I don't know.*
> Alzheimer: *It's difficult, isn't it?*
> Auguste D: *So anxious, so anxious.*

In another interview, he asks her to write her name. She can't get beyond Mrs, even with prompting, and repeats: 'Ich hab mich verloren.' (I have lost myself.)

What was so special about Auguste D's case that drove Alzheimer to spend years on researching, then presenting it at a European meeting?

Auguste D was only forty-nine when her descent into a bizarre form of dementia began, so rapid that she was dead by the age of fifty-seven. This was no age related decline in mental agility.

The microscopic changes in the brain that Alzheimer found at post-mortem were equally bizarre – the like of which nobody had seen before. There were protein plaques and tangled filaments choking the brain cells so much that the brain was shrunken (cerebral atrophy) like Carl's was. Alzheimer also noted atherosclerosis (furring up) in the brain arteries which Anitschow would confidently state in 1913 could not occur without cholesterol – as we saw in Chapter 17. But Alzheimer's colleague, Perusini, didn't agree, thus anticipating the debates on the aetiology and management of dementia syndromes that would preoccupy researchers and clinicians from the second half of the twentieth century onwards.

Glossary and Abbreviations

Adv Psych Treatment – Advances in Psychiatric Treatment

aetiology – the cause of a disease

affective disorder – any psychiatric disorder featuring disturbances of mood or emotion

Ageing Res Rev – Ageing Research Reviews

Allg. Z. Psychiat – Allgemeine Zeitschrift für Psychiatrie

Alzheimer's disease – the commonest form of dementia characterised by recent memory loss and at brain biopsy or post mortem by protein deposits and tangles in the brain

Am J Alzheimers Dis Other Demen – American Journal of Alzheimer's Disease and Other Dementias

Am J Clin Nutr – The American Journal of Clinical Nutrition

Am J Epidemiol – The American Journal of Epidemiology

Arch Gen Psych – Archives of General Psychiatry

Arch Neurol – Archives of Neurology

arteriole – a small branch of an artery leading into many smaller vessels, the capillaries

artery – a blood vessel carrying blood away from the heart

arteriosclerosis – an imprecise term used for any of several conditions affecting the arteries. The term is often used as a synonym for atherosclerosis

atheroma – degeneration of the walls of the arteries due to the formation in them of fatty plaques and scar tissue

atherosclerosis – a disease of the arteries in which fatty plaques develop on their inner walls with eventual obstruction of blood flow

atrophy – the wasting away of a normally developed organ or tissue due to degeneration of cells

Aust NZ J Psychiatry – Australian and New Zealand Journal of Psychiatry

axon – a nerve fibre extending from the main body of the *neuron* or nerve cell

BJGP – British Journal of General Practice

BJP – British Journal of Psychiatry

Bratisl Lek Listy – Bratislavské lekárske listy (Bratislava Medical Journal)

BMJ – British Medical Journal

central nervous system – the brain and spinal cord

cerebrum (adj. cerebral) – the largest and most highly developed part of the brain consisting of the two cerebral hemispheres each with an outer layer of *grey matter*, the cerebral cortex, responsible for perception, memory, thought, and intellect. It is divided into functional regions

cholesterol – a fat like material (sterol) present in the blood and most tissues, especially nervous tissue; high levels of 'bad' LDL-cholesterol in the blood are related to *atheroma*

CMAJ – Canadian Medical Association Journal

cognition (adj. cognitive as in cognitive impairment) – thinking or intellectual functioning: memory, planning, reasoning, language, numeracy, attention, and visuo-spatial awareness

cohort (longitudinal) study – a systematic study of a group of people which may be conducted retrospectively (examining data relating to the group's history of exposure and disease experience) or prospectively (systematically following up subjects for a defined period of time or until the occurrence of a specified event)

Curr Treat Options Neurol – Current Treatment Options in Neurology

dementia – a chronic and progressive deterioration of behaviour and higher intellectual function due to organic brain disease. It is marked by memory disorders, changes in personality, impaired reasoning ability and disorientation

dyslipidaemia – abnormality of blood fat e.g. raised cholesterol

EBM – Endocrinology, Biochemistry and Metabolism

ECR – European Court Reports

Eur Heart J – Eurpoean Heart Journal

embolus (adj. embolic as in *embolic stroke*) – material, such as a blood clot, that is carried by the blood from one point in the circulation to lodge at another point

epidemiology – the study of the distribution in populations of diseases and their determinants

Eur J Epidemiol – European Journal of Epidemiology

executive function – the co-ordination in the pre-frontal cerebral cortex, immediately behind the forehead, of other cognitive processes: working memory, attention, reasoning, planning and problem solving

fraternal (dizygotic) twins – result from simultaneous fertilization of two egg cells therefore not necessarily of same gender and no more alike than siblings from separate pregnancies. Compare *identical (monozygotic) twins*

functional disorder – a condition in which a patient complains of symptoms for which no physical cause can be found. Such a condition may be an indication of a psychiatric disorder. Compare *organic disorder*

grey matter – the darker coloured tissues of the central nervous system composed mainly of the cell bodies of *neurons*

hyperlipidaemia – raised levels of circulating blood fats e.g. cholesterol, and triglycerides

hypertension – raised blood pressure

identical (monozygotic) twins – result from fertilization of a single egg cell that subsequently divides to form two separate foetuses. Compare *fraternal (dizygotic) twins*

ischaemia – inadequate flow of blood to the body part in question

JAMA – Journal of the American Medical Association

JACN – Journal of the American College of Nutrition

JCEM – The Journal of Clinical Endocrinology & Metabolism

J Neurol Neurosurg Psych – Journal of Neurology, Neurosurgery & Psychiatry

Med Clin North Am – Medical Clinics of North America

Med Leg J – Medico-Legal Journal

multi-infarct dementia – a type of vascular dementia due to the destruction of brain tissue by a series of small strokes

NEJM – New England Journal of Medicine

NIH – National Institutes of Health

neuron – the basic functional unit, the nerve cell, of the *central nervous system*

neurologist – a specialist in the structure, functioning and diseases of the nervous system

NHSE – National Health Service Executive

organic disorder – a condition associated with changes in the structure of an organ or tissue. Compare *functional disorder*

pathology – the study of disease processes by examination of samples e.g. blood from living patients or at autopsy. Hence neuro-pathology, the study of the nervous system and chemical pathology, the study of disordered body chemistry

peer review – the assessment by appropriate experts, on behalf of the editor of an academic journal, of the quality and validity of an article submitted for publication

plaque – a deposit with a fatty core that develops in the inner wall of an artery in atherosclerosis

Postgrad Med J – Postgraduate Medical Journal

Proc Nutr Soc – Proceedings of the Nutrition Society

primary prevention – avoidance of the onset of disease by behaviour modification or treatment

psychiatrist – a medically qualified specialist in the study and treatment of mental disorders

psychologist – a person engaged in the scientific study of the mind

randomised controlled trial, RCT – a comparison of the outcome between two or more groups of patients that are deliberately subjected to different regimes to test a hypothesis, usually of treatment. Entrants to the trial are allocated to their respective groups by random numbers. In a double blind trial neither patients nor observers know the group to which the patient has been assigned

Recenti Prog Med – Recenti Progressi in Medicina

risk factor – something that increases a person's chance of developing a condition

secondary prevention – the avoidance or alleviation of disease by early detection and appropriate management

sign – an indication of a disorder that is found by a doctor when examining a patient. Compare *symptom*

stroke – damage to an area of the brain caused by interruption of the blood flow to it or bleeding into it. The cause may be *thrombotic* (blockage in a damaged blood vessel), *embolic* (blockage caused by broken-off blood clot formed elsewhere in the body) or haemorrhagic (ruptured blood vessel causing bleeding into the brain tissue as may occur in *hypertension*)

symptom – an indication of a disease or disorder noticed by the patient. A presenting symptom is one that leads the patient to consult a doctor. Compare *sign*

TATT – common medical acronym for 'tired all the time'

tertiary prevention – reducing the impact of complications and progression of established disease

thrombosis, adj. thrombotic – thrombus (blood clot) formation within the blood vessels as can occur in disorders of the blood and blood vessels

triglyceride – a circulating blood fat, raised levels of which can lead to arterial blockage

UKSC – United Kingdom Supreme Court

vascular – relating to blood vessels

vascular dementia – dementia in which damage to the brain tissue is caused by impaired blood supply through ruptured or blocked blood vessels

References

Chapter 2
1. The Slaughterhouses (Hygiene) and Meat Inspection (Amendment) Regulations 1991, No. 984 [enactment date 13th May 1991].

Chapter 7
2. Alzheimer's drug gets the go-ahead. *Daily Mail,* 26 February, 1997.

Chapter 12
3. Bhatnagar, D. and Durrington, P. N. (1989). Borderline hypercholesterolaemia: when to introduce drugs. *Postgrad Med J* 65(766):543-552.
4. The Slaughterhouses (Hygiene) and Meat Inspection (Amendment) Regulations 1991, No. 984 Op cit. Chapter 2.

Chapter 14
5. Alzheimer's drug gets the go-ahead. *Daily Mail,* 26 February, 1997. Op cit. Chapter 7.

Chapter 15
6. NHS Executive (1996). *Complaints: Listening...Acting... Improving: Guidance on Implementation of the NHS Complaints Procedure.* Leeds: NHSE.
7. Brazier, M. (2003). *Medicine, Patients and the Law.* 3rd ed. London: Penguin Books Ltd.

Chapter 16

8.   Small, G.W. *et al* (1997). Diagnosis and treatment of Alzheimer disease and related disorders: consensus statement of the American Association for Geriatric Psychiatry, the Alzheimer's Association and the American Geriatrics Society. *JAMA,* 278(16):1363-1371.

9.   Williams, I. (1994). Chapter 10 Older People. In: Pullen, I. et al, (eds.) *Psychiatry and General Practice Today.* London: Royal College of Psychiatrists and Royal College of General Practitioners.

10.   Rabins, P.V. (1983). Reversible dementia and the misdiagnosis of dementia: a review. *Hosp Community Psychiatry* 34(9):830-835.

Chapter 17

11.   Durrington, P.N. (1989). *Hyperlipidaemia Diagnosis and Treatment.* Sevenoaks: Wright (imprint of Butterworth Scientific).

12.   Fisher, C.M. (1968). Dementia in cerebral vascular disease. In: Tools, J.F. et al, (eds) *Cerebral vascular diseases, 6th Conference,* Grune New York:232-236. Cited by Hachinsky (1992) in ref. 15.

13.   Block, W. (2008). Galantamine Benefits Both Alzheimer's Disease and Vascular Dementia. lifeenhancement.com/magazine/January/2008

14.   Hachinsky, V.C. *et al* (1974). Multi-infarct dementia a cause of mental deterioration in the elderly. *Lancet* 1974 (ii):207-210.

15.   Hachinsky, V.C. (1992). Preventable senility: a call for action against the vascular dementias. *Lancet* 340:645-648.

16.   International Network of Cholesterol Skeptics. thincs.org

17.   Bhatnagar, D. & Durrington, P.N. (1989). Op. cit. Chapter 12, ref. 3.

Chapter 18

18.   Hofman, A. *et al* (1991). Determinants of disease and disability in the elderly: the Rotterdam elderly study. *Eur J Epidemiol* 7(4):403-422.

19. Gruetzner, H. (1992). *Alzheimer's: a caregiver's guide and sourcebook*. New York: John Wiley and Sons, Inc.

20. Heilman, K.M. and Fisher, W.R. (1974). Hyperlipidemic dementia. *Arch Neurol* 31(7):67-68.

21. Hachinsky, V.C. (1992). Op. cit. Chapter 17, ref. 15.

22. Nolan, K.A. and Blass, J.P. (1992). Preventing cognitive decline. *Clinics in Geriatric Medicine*, 8(1):19-34.

23. Stewart, R. *et al* (1999). Vascular risk factors and Alzheimer's disease. *Aust NZ J Psychiatry* 33(6):809-813.

24. Skoog, I. (1994). Risk factors for vascular dementia: a review. *Dementia* 5(3-4):137-144.

25. Amar, K. and Wilcock, G. (1996). Fortnightly Review: Vascular dementia. *BMJ* 312:227-231.

26. De Deyn, P.P. *et al* (1999). From neuronal and vascular impairment to dementia. *Pharmacopsychiatry* 32, Suppl1:17-24.

27. Harvey, Fox and Rossor (1999). *Dementia Handbook*. London: Martin Dunitz.

28. Davidson, E.A. and Robertson, E.E. (1955). Alzheimer's disease with acne roseacea in one of identical twins. *J Neurol Neurosurg Psych* 1872-1877.

29. Renvoize, E.B. *et al* (1986). Identical twins discordant for presenile dementia of the Alzheimer type. *Brit J Psych* 149:509-512.

30. Kumar, A. *et al* (1991). Anatomic, metabolic, neuropsychological, and molecular genetic studies of three pairs of identical twins discordant for dementia of the Alzheimer's type. *Arch Neurol* 48(2):160-68.

31. Gatz, M. *et al* (1997). Heritability for Alzheimer's disease: the study of dementia in Swedish twins. *J Gerontol A Biol Sci Med Sci* 52A(2): 117-125.

32. Bergem, A.L.M. *et al* (1997). The role of heredity in late-onset Alzheimer disease and vascular dementia: a twin study. *Arch Gen Psychiatry* 54(3):264-270.

33. Hardy, J. The role of genetics in Alzheimer's. HBO Documentary Films for the Alzheimer's Association.

alz.org/research/video/video_pages/genetics_in_alz.html

34. Fratiglioni, L. *et al* (2000). Incidence of dementia and major subtypes in Europe: a collaborative study of population-based cohorts. *Neurology* 54 (11 Suppl 5): S10-15.

35. Ortega, R.M. *et al* (1997). Dietary intake and cognitive function in a group of elderly people. *Am J Clin Nutr* 66(4):803-809.

36. Solfrizzi, V. (1999). High monounsaturated fatty acids intake protects against age-related cognitive decline. *Neurology* 52(8):1563.

37. The Harvard Medical School (2007). *The truth about fats: bad and good.* Family Health Guide. health.harvard.educ/fhg/updates/Truth-about-fats.shtml

38. Bhatnagar, D. & Durrington, P.N. (1989). Op. cit. Chapter 12, ref. 3.

Chapter 19

39. Gruetzner, H. (1992). Op. cit. Chapter 18, ref. 19.

Chapter 26

40. Bhatnagar, D. & Durrington, P.N. (1989). Op.cit. Chapter 12, ref. 3.

41. Q Risk score. qrisk.org

Chapter 28

42. Merry, A. & Smith, A.McC. (2001). Chapter 7 Assessing the standard – the role of the expert witness. *Errors, Medicine and the Law.* Cambridge: University Press.

Chapter 37

43. McCullagh, C.D. *et al* (2001). Risk factors for dementia. *Adv Psych Treatment* 7:24-31.

44. Pericak-Vance, M.A. & Haines, J.L. (1995). Genetic susceptibility to Alzheimer's disease. *Trends in Genetics* 11: 504-508. Cited by McCullough *et al, ibid.*

45. Hachinsky, V.C. (1992). Op.cit. Chapter 17, ref. 15.

46. Amar, K. and Wilcock, G. (1996). Op.cit. Chapter 18, ref. 25.

47. Harvey, Fox and Rossor (1999). Op.cit. Chapter 18, ref. 27.
48. Gruetzner, H. (1992). Op.cit. Chapter 18, ref. 19.

Chapter 40

49. The Right Honourable the Lord Woolf, Master of the Rolls, July 1996 Access to Justice: Final Report to the Lord Chancellor on the civil justice system in England and Wales.
50. Statutory Instrument (1998). *Access to Justice. The Civil Procedure Rules 1998*, No. 332 (L.17).

Chapter 46

51. Beare, S. (2005). *50 Secrets of the World's Longest Living People*. New York: Marlowe & Co.
52. Minicocci, I. *et al* (2013). Mutations in the ANGPTL3 gene and familial combined hypolipidaemia. *JCEM* 97(7):1266-1275.
53. Cugini, P. *et al* (1995). The Campodimele Study: 24-hour blood pressure in rural life-style subjects. *Recenti Prog Med* 86(7-8):265-271 [English abstract].
54. Willcox, B.J., Willcox, C.D. & Suzuki, M. (2001). *The Okinawa Way* London: Mermaid Books.
55. Hughes, T.F. *et al* (2010). Midlife fruit and vegetable consumption and risk of dementia in later life in Swedish twins. *Am J Ger Psych* 18(5):413-420.
56. Xu, W.L. *et al* (2011). Midlife overweight and obesity increase late-life dementia risk: a population-based twin study. *Neurology* 76(18): 1568-1574.
57. Morris, M.C. (2009). The role of nutrition in Alzheimer's disease: epidemiological evidence. *Eur J Neurol* 16(Suppl.1):1-7.
58. Bowler, J.V. and Hachinski, V. (eds) (2003). *Vascular Cognitive Impairment: preventable dementia*. New York: Oxford University Press.
59. Sparks, D.L. *et al* (2005). Atorvastatin for the treatment of mild to moderate Alzheimer disease: preliminary results. *Arch Neurol* 62:753-757.

60. Masse, I. *et al* (2005). Lipid lowering agents are associated with a lower cognitive decline in Alzheimer's disease. *J Neurol Neurosurg Psychiatry* 76:1624-1629.

61. Deschaintre, Y. *et al* (2009). Treatment of vascular risk factors is associated with slower decline in Alzheimer's disease. *Neurology* 73(9):674-680.

62. Etminan, M. *et al* (2003). The role of lipid lowering drugs in cognitive function: a meta-analysis of observational studies. *Pharmacotherapy* 23(6):726-730.

63. Stewart, R. *et al* (1999). Op. cit. Chapter 18, ref. 23.

64. Inzitari, D., Lamassa, M. & Pantoni, L. (2003). Treatment of vascular dementia. In: Bowler, J.V. and Hachinski, V (eds.) *Vascular Cognitive Impairment: preventable dementia.* Op cit. Chapter 46, ref.58, 277-292.

65. Marler, J. (2003). Clinical trials in vascular dementia. In: Bowler, J.V. and Hachinski, V (eds.) *Vascular Cognitive Impairment: preventable dementia.* Op cit. Chapter 46, ref.58. 293-307.

66. Gorelick, P.B. (2003). Prevention. In: Bowler, J.V. and Hachinski, V (eds.) *Vascular Cognitive Impairment: preventable dementia.* Op cit. Chapter 46, ref.58, 308-321.

67. Kivipelto, M. *et al* (2001). Midlife vascular risk factors and Alzheimer's disease in later life: longitudinal, population based study. *BMJ* 322:1447.

68. Meyer, J.S. et al. (1986). Improved cognition after control of risk factors for multi-infarct dementia. *JAMA* 256(16):2203-2209.

69. Richard, F. and Pasquier, F. (2012). Can the treatment of vascular risk factors slow cognitive decline in Alzheimer's disease patients? *J Alzheimers Dis* 32:765-772.

70. Ducharme, F. *et al* (2013). The unique experience of spouses in early-onset dementia. *Am J Alzheimers Dis Other Demen* 28(6):634-41.

71. Pasquier, F. (2013). Young Onset Alzheimer's Disease. youtube.com/watch? v=Gb6rLtJkS8g uploaded by Dementia Services Ireland.

72. Purandara, N. and Burns, A. (2005). Vascular Dementia Factsheet. pssru.ac.uk/pdf/MCpdfs/Vascular_dementia_factsheet_2005.pdf

73. National Institute for Health and Clinical Excellence (2013). *National Clinical Practice Guideline Number 42* Leicester: The British Psychological Society.

74. Alzheimer's Society (2013). Factsheet 402: What is Vascular Dementia?

75. Vascular dementia (2013). *BMJ* Best Practice. bestpractice.bmj.com/best-practice/monograph/319/resources.html

Chapter 47

76. Brennan, T., Leape, L., Laird, N. *et al* (1991). Incidence of adverse events and negligence in hospitalized patients: the results from the Harvard Medical Practice Study I, *NEJM* 324:370-376.

77. Brennan, T., Leape, L., Laird, N. *et al* (1991). Incidence of adverse events and negligence in hospitalized patients: the results from the Harvard Medical Practice Study II, *NEJM* 324:377-84.

Chapter 48

78. Brennan, T., Leape, L., Laird, N. *et al* (1991). Op.cit. Chapter 47, ref. 76.

79. Brennan, T., Leape, L., Laird, N. *et al* (1991). Op.cit. Chapter 47, ref. 77.

80. Watkins, S. (1987). *Medicine and Labour: the Politics of a Profession.* London: Lawrence and Wishart.

81. Daniels, B. (2010). *Confessions of a GP.* London: Harper Collins.

82. Riley, P. (1992). *Serious Misconduct.* London: Robert Hale Ltd.

Chapter 49

83. Harrison, S. (2013). Have you got the right leg? How to avoid 'wrong-site' surgery. *FT Weekend Magazine,* 14/15 September, p.50.

84. Rosenthal, M.M. *et al* (1999). *Medical Mishaps Pieces of the Puzzle.* Buckingham: Open University Press.

85. Leape, L.L. (1999). Chapter 2 Error in medicine. In: *Medical Mishaps Pieces of the puzzle*. Buckingham: Open University Press.

86. Brennan, T., Leape, L., Laird, N. *et al.* (1991). Op. cit. Chapter 47, ref. 76.

87. Brennan, T., Leape, L., Laird, N. *et al.* (1991). Op. cit. Chapter 47, ref. 77.

88. Vincent, C. and Reason, J. (1999). Chapter 3 Human Factors Approaches in Medicine. In: *Medical Mishaps Pieces of the puzzle*. Buckingham: Open University Press.

89. Sheen, Mr Justice (1987). *MV Herald of Free Enterprise. Report of Court No. 8074. Formal Investigation*. London: Department of Transport.

90. Bromiley, M. (2007). Just a Routine Operation: human factors in patient safety. NHS Institute for Innovation and Improvement. youtube.com/watch?v=jzlvgtPIof4

91. Giddings, T. (2007). Just a Routine Operation. youtube.com/watch?v=lEbMKgiSlvc

Chapter 50

92. Batt, J. (2004). *Stolen Innocence.* London: Random House.

93. Watkins, S.J. (2000). Conviction by mathematical error? *BMJ* 320(7226): 2-3.

94. The Royal Statistical Society (2001). Statement regarding statistical issues in the Sally Clark case. 23 October. therss.org.uk/archive/sclark.html

Chapter 51

95. Simpson, K. (1984). *Forty Years of Murder.* London: Book Club Associates.

96. Bowen, D. (2003). *Body of Evidence.* London: Constable & Robinson Ltd.

97. Rose, A. (2007). *Lethal Witness.* Stroud: Sutton Publishing.

98. Smith, S. *Mostly Murder.* 3rd ed. London: Panther Books.

99. The 'Woolf report'. Op. cit. Chapter 40, ref. 49.

100. The 'Woolf reforms'. Op. cit. Chapter 40, ref. 50.
101. Watkins, S. (1987). Op. cit. Chapter 48, ref. 80.
102. *Jones v Kaney* Supreme Court decision (30 March 2011) UKSC 13.

Chapter 52
103. Lewis, C. J. (2006) 6th ed. *Clinical Negligence: a practical guide.* Haywards Heath: Tottel Publishing.
104. Rosenthal, M.M., Mulcahy, L. and Lloyd-Bostock, S. (1999). *Medical Mishaps Pieces of the puzzle.* Op. cit. Chapter 49, ref. 84.
105. Watkins, S. (1987). Op. cit. Chapter 48, ref. 80.
106. Mulcahy, L. *et al* (1999). *Mediating Medical Negligence Claims: An option for the future?* London: The Stationery Office.
107. NHS Executive (1996). Op. cit. Chapter 15, ref. 6.
108. Allen, M.T. (2005) A new way to settle old disputes. *Med Leg J* 73(3):93-110.

Chapter 54
109. Dickens, M. (1952). *One Pair of Feet.* London: Mermaid Books.
110. Durrington, P.N. *Hyperlipidaemia Diagnosis and Treatment.* Op. cit. Chapter 17, ref. 11.
111. Working Group on Lipoprotein Measurement (1995). *Recommendations on Lipoprotein Measurement.* NIH publication No. 95-3044.
112. Porter, M. (2014). Q A. *Times 2,* 25 February, p.6.
113. Porter, M. (2014). Statins could save your life but these are the risks you must know about. *Times 2,* 25 March, p.6.
114. Powell v The United Kingdom (2004). *European Court of Human Rights* ECR 3rd Section, 4 May Application No. 45305/99. hudoc. echr.coe.int/sites/eng/pages/search.aspx?i=001-5215

Chapter 55
115. Mapstone, M. (2014). *Nature Medicine* 20:415-418.
116. O'Connor, D.W. *et al* (1993). Dementia in general practice:

the practical consequences of a more positive approach to diagnosis. *BJGP* 43:185-188.

Postscript

117. Alzheimer, A. (1899). Beitrag zur pathologischen Anatomie der Seelenstörungen des Greisenhalters. *Allg. Z. Psychiat* 56:272-273. (English translation by Hans Förstl and Barbara Beats).
118. Alzheimer, A. (1906). In: Maurer, K. *et al* (1997). Auguste D and Alzheimer's disease. *Lancet* 349:1546-1549.
119. Maurer, K. and Maurer, U. (1998). *Alzheimer The Life of a Physician and the Career of a Disease.* München: Piper Verlag GmbH. English translation by Neil Levi with Alistair Burns (2003). New York: Columbia University Press.
120. Graeber, M.B. (2005). In: Zilka, N. & Novak, M. (2006). The tangled story of Alois Alzheimer. *Bratisl Lek Listv* 107(9-10):343-345.

Bibliography

Because this is not a comprehensive review of the literature, I have included only those landmark publications uncited in the text which emphasise that the now widespread recognition of the role of modifiable risk factors for dementia, including Alzheimer type, had begun in specialist units some years before Carl Valente's dementing illness began.

Kral, V.A. (1962). Senescent forgetfulness: benign and malignant. *CMAJ* 86(6):257-260.

Cummings, J. *et al* (1980). Reversible dementia: illustrative cases, definition and review. *JAMA* 243(23):2434-2439.

Cummings, J., Benson, D.F. and LoVerne, S. (1983). *Dementia: a clinical approach.* Oxford: Butterworth-Heinemann.

Mueller, J. et al (1983). Hyperviscosity induced dementia. Neurology 31(1):101.

Meyer, J.S. *et al* (1988). Aetiological consideration and risk factors for multi-infarct dementia. *J Neurol Neurosurg Psych* 51:1489-1497.

Meyer, J.S. *et al* (1989). Randomized clinical trial of daily aspirin in multi-infarct dementia: a pilot study. *J Am Geriatr Soc* 37(6):549-555.

Hachinski, V.C. (1990). The decline and resurgence of vascular dementia. *CMAJ* 142(2):107-111.

Hofman, A. *et al* (1991). Determinants of disease and disability in the elderly: the Rotterdam elderly study. *Eur J Epidemiol* 7(4):403-422.

Jama, J.W. (1996). Dietary anti-oxidants and cognitive function in a population-based sample of older persons: the Rotterdam Study. *Am J Epidemiol* 144(3):275-280.

Hofman, A. *et al* (1997). Atherosclerosis, Apolipoprotein E, and prevalence of dementia and Alzheimer's disease in the Rotterdam study. *Lancet* 349:151-154.

Kalmijn, S. *et al* (1997). Dietary fat intake and the risk of incident dementia in the Rotterdam Study. *Ann Neurol* 42:776-782.

Snowdon, D.A. *et al* (1997). Brain infarction and the clinical expression of Alzheimer disease: the Nun Study. *JAMA* 277(10):813-817.

Breteler, M.M.B. *et al* (1998). Risk factors for vascular disease and dementia. *Haemostasis* 28:167-173.

Forette, F. *at al* (1998). Prevention of dementia in randomised double-blind placebo-controlled Systolic Hypertension in Europe (Syst-Eur) trial. *Lancet* 352(9137):1347-51.

Petersen, R.C. (1999). Mild cognitive impairment. *Arch Neurol* 56:303-308.

Moroney, J.T. *et al* (1999). Low-density lipoprotein cholesterol and the risk of dementia with stroke. *JAMA* 281(3):254-260.

Selkoe, D.J. (1999). Review: Translating cell biology into therapeutic advances in Alzheimer's disease. *Nature* 399 Suppl:23-31.

Jick, H. *et al* (2000). Statins and the risk of dementia. *Lancet* 356:1627-1631.

Devasenapathy, A. and Hachinsky, V.C. (2000). Vascular cognitive impairment. *Curr Treat Options Neurol* 2(1):61-72.

Wolozin, B. *et al* (2000). Decreased prevalence of Alzheimer disease associated with 3-hydroxy-3-methylglutaryl coenzyme A reductase inhibitors. *Arch Neurol* 57(10):1439-1443.

Rogers, P.J. (2001). A healthy body, a healthy mind: long-term impact of diet on mood and cognitive function. *Proc Nutr Soc* 60(1):135-143.

Román, G.C. (2002). Vascular dementia revisited: diagnosis, pathogenesis, treatment, and prevention. *Med Clin North Am* 86(3):477-99.

Launer, L.J. (2002). Demonstrating the case that Alzheimer's disease is a vascular disease: epidemiologic evidence. *Ageing Res Rev* 1(1):61-77.

O'Brien, J.T. *et al* (2003). *Lancet* 2(2):89-98.

Wolozin, B. (2004). Cholesterol and the biology of Alzheimer's disease. Mini review. *Neuron* 41: 7-10.

Erkinjuntti, T. *et al* (2004). Emerging therapies for vascular dementia and vascular cognitive impairment. *Stroke* 35:1010-1017.

Winblad, B. *et al* (2004). Mild cognitive impairment – beyond controversies, towards a consensus: report of the International Working Group on mild cognitive impairment. Key symposium. *J Int Med* 256:240-246.

Burke, D. *et al* (2007). Possibilities for the prevention and treatment of cognitive impairment and dementia. *BJP* 190:371-372.

Alagiskrishnan, K. *et al* (2008). Treating vascular risk factors and maintaining vascular health: is this the way towards successful cognitive ageing and preventing cognitive decline? *Postgrad Med J* 82(964):101-105.

Murray, I.V.J. *et al* (2011). Vascular and metabolic dysfunction in Alzheimer's disease: a review. *EBM* 236:772-782.

Kaffashian, S. *et al* (2011). Predictive utility of the Framingham general cardiovascular disease risk profile for cognitive function: evidence from the Whitehall II study. *Eur Heart J* 32:2326-2332.

Alzheimer's Society (2012). Am I at risk of developing dementia? Factsheet 350.

Martin, E.A. (2010) ed. *Oxford Concise Medical Dictionary*. Oxford: University Press.

Useful Organisations

Alzheimer's Society – Help and information on all aspects of dementia
Devon House
58 St Katharine's Way
London E1W 1LB
020 7423 3500
Helpline: 0300 222 11 22
enquiries@alzheimers.org.uk
alzheimers.org.uk

Mind– Mental health charity
15–19 Broadway
Stratford
London E15 4BQ
020 8519 2122
Helpline: 0300 123 3393 or text 86463
contact@mind.org.uk
mind.org.uk

SANDS – Stillbirths and neonatal deaths charity
28 Portland Place
London
W1B 1LY
020 7436 7940
Helpline: 020 7436 5881
helpline@uk-sands.org
uk-sands.org

The Patients Association– Patients' rights charity
PO Box 935
Harrow
Middlesex
HA1 3YJ
020 8423 9111
Helpline: 0845 608 4455
helpline@patients-association.com
mailbox@patients-association.com
patients-association.com

About the Author

Renata Payne is a retired specialist in laboratory medicine.

Lightning Source UK Ltd.
Milton Keynes UK
UKOW04f0734250315

248489UK00003B/63/P